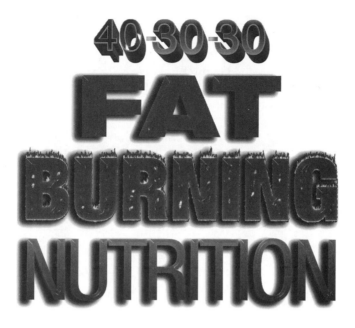

40·30·30 FAT BURNING NUTRITION

The Dietary Hormonal Connection to Permanent Weight Loss and Better Health

by Joyce & Gene Daoust

Wharton Publishing
Del Mar, California

The information contained in this book is from the authors' experiences and is not intended to replace medical advice. The authors do not directly or indirectly dispense medical advice or prescribe the use of this nutritional program as a form of treatment.

This publication is presented for information purposes, to increase public knowledge of the developments in the field of nutrition. Before beginning this or any nutrition program you should consult with your physician, and address any questions to your physician.

Use of the information provided is at the sole choice and risk of the reader.

Library of Congress Catalog Card Number 96-61472
Publisher's Cataloging-in-Publication
        (Prepared by Quality Books, Inc.)

Daoust, Joyce.
    40-30-30 fat-burning nutrition: the dietary hormonal connection to permanent weight loss and better health/Joyce and Gene Daoust.
    p. cm.
    ISBN: 1-56912-086-2
    1. Reducing diets.   2. Nutrition.
    I. Daoust, Gene.   II. Title.   III. Title: Forty-thirty-thirty fat-burning nutrition.
RM222.2.D36 1996   6.13.2'5
                               QBI96-20509

EDITOR .... Peter Economy – San Diego, California
CONTRIBUTING EDITOR .... Christine Paffrath – Dixon, California
COVER DESIGN .... Carolyn Seligson – Encinitas, California
LAYOUT DESIGN/PRODUCTION ..... Kara Meredith, Creative Services – Oceanside, California

PRINTED IN THE UNITED STATES OF AMERICA

Dedication

This book is dedicated to and in memory of Gene's parents, Donald J. and Mary Jean Daoust, for being such wonderful teachers and great friends. You may be gone but will never be forgotten, and I will always "Keep the Faith and Think Big."

This book is also dedicated to Joyce's parents, Richard and Clarann Ruhmann, for giving her the strength and independence to overcome any obstacle and accomplish any goal.

Table of Contents

Biography

JOYCE AND GENE DAOUST

Married for 10 years, Joyce and Gene Daoust continue to marry their talents as managing editors of *Fat-Burning Nutrition News*, a quarterly newsletter dedicated entirely to *Fat-Burning Nutrition*, and as president and director, respectively, of FBN Enterprises, their nutritional consulting firm located in San Diego, California. As former directors and co-founders of the Bio-Syn Human Performance Center, a cutting-edge weight loss and sports nutrition clinic in Redmond, Washington, they were key members of the original clinical nutrition team that developed the 40-30-30 diet—a diet based on hormonal responses to foods.

Moving theory into practice, the Daousts developed the nutrition programs for three start-up companies that make 40-30-30 meal replacement nutrition bars. Having conducted thousands of nutritional and body fat analyses, Joyce and Gene also created *The Two-Week Fat Flush*, a simple and fast weight loss program, and *The Corporate Executive Fat Loss Challenge*, a weight loss and performance nutrition program for corporations.

Gene is a certified nutritionist and former bodybuilder. He has come to be known as *"The Amino Man,"* because of his expertise in the areas of amino acids, weight loss, sports nutrition, and dietary endocrinology.

Joyce is also a certified nutritionist and has prepared personalized nutrition plans and worked with physicians to help thousands of people eat well while burning fat. Joyce is also the co-host of "Fitness Awareness," a weekly radio program that discusses the latest in exercise, fat-burning nutrition, and how anyone can look, feel, and perform better.

Joyce and Gene have become leading speakers at seminars and workshops for the general public, health food industry, corporations and health professionals, and have working relationships with many professional athletes and teams. They are also featured columnists, weight loss advisors, and contributing editors for numerous health and fitness newsletters and magazines.

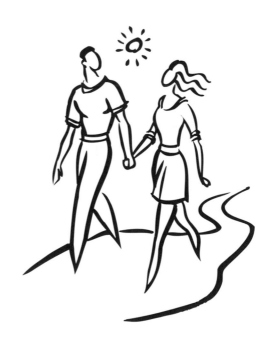

Introduction

NUTRITIONIST DISCOVERS HOW YOU CAN MAXIMIZE YOUR BODY'S ABILITY TO BURN STORED BODY FAT 24 HOURS A DAY, EVERYDAY!

Sound like a crazy headline from a tabloid magazine, too good to be true? Maybe, but it *is* true, and right now as you read this, you should be burning stored body fat for energy. In fact, if you ate the right balance of carbohydrate, protein, and fat in your last meal, you would have no choice but to burn fat for energy. You see, every time you eat you have the ability to control the hormones that burn fat and store fat in your body. These hormones are controlled by the balance of the macronutrients that are found in the foods you eat. You have the ability to control these hormones every time you eat, 24 hours a day, *every* day.

If, like most people, you have been following the high-carbohydrate, low- or fat-free recommendations of the so-called experts, you probably are not burning stored body fat as efficiently as possible but are burning sugars (carbohydrates) instead.

The so-called experts are WRONG! You see, there is a big difference in weight loss diets and

40-30-30 Fat-Burning Nutrition. The secret is balanced nutrition. It always has been and always will be. The high-carbohydrate and low- or fat-free approach is *not* balanced and is hormonally incorrect to burn fat. The current advice that says "a calorie is a calorie, simply reduce your calories or exercise like crazy" does not tell the whole story. To maximize fat burning, it's not what you eat that is important, but the *balance* of what you eat and the hormonal response it creates.

All of this talk about balanced hormones is the result of understanding a little known specialty called dietary endocrinology, the study of how foods affect hormonal response. This book offers an optimal eating program based on a 40-30-30 ratio of carbohydrate, protein, and fat which we used exclusively at the BioSyn Human Performance Center in Seattle, Washington.

> To maximize fat burning, it's not what you eat, but the *balance* of what you eat and the hormonal response created, that is important.

40-30-30 Fat-Burning Nutrition is simple to use, safe, and easy to get started. Our system is complete, and it provides clear and concise direction on how to maximize your body's ability to burn stored body fat.

We have accumulated over 25 years of combined experience in the fields of fat and weight loss, sports nutrition, and performance nutrition and have seen the *40-30-30* program work for more than 50,000 people. We *know* it can work for you. Keep your fat burning hope alive, good luck, keep the faith, and just burn it. Fat that is!

Gene and Joyce Daoust

How to Use This Book

THIS BOOK IS FOR YOU

> • If you are too fat
> • If you crave sugars or carbohydrates
> • If you have been following a high-carbohydrate, low-fat diet and are not losing body fat
> • If you are sick and tired of fad diets that don't work

Why? Because 95 percent of all diets fail. Americans are eating less fat and more carbohydrates and are now fatter than ever!

And... because it's time to understand the true science behind nutrition—specifically the dietary hormonal connection to *40-30-30 Fat-Burning Nutrition.*

HOW THIS BOOK CAN HELP YOU

We have organized *40-30-30 Fat-Burning Nutrition* from the point of view of one who likes to read and understand a concept thoroughly before he tries it out. However, you might prefer to skip the scientific background presented in the first section and get to the "hands-on" part of the program, so you can begin to burn fat right away. You can always come back to the first section and take your time learning about the scientific background that is the basis for the program. We hope that, whichever method you choose, you will enjoy and become excited about making *40-30-30 Fat-Burning Nutrition* a part of your life.

Following is a brief synopsis of each section of the book to help you decide the best way to begin.

Part I

Chapters 1 through 5 take you on a simplified scientific journey to understanding how your body works and what happens hormonally when you eat certain kinds of foods. We have tried to use familiar vocabulary and to define terms that may be new to non-scientists, which most of us are. These chapters deal with how your intake of carbohydrate, protein, and fat control the two major hormones that determine how efficiently you burn stored body fat for energy. You will find out that, by using a specific 40-30-30 ratio of carbohydrate, protein, and fat at each meal, you have the ability to control the fat storage hormone and the fat burning hormones every time you eat.

Although you can lose body fat by following *40-30-30 Fat-Burning Nutrition* alone, Chapter 3 points out the hormonal benefits of adding some exercise to your life. The additional health benefits to be gained from burning stored body fat are discussed in Chapter 6.

Part II

Chapter 7 offers a vegetarian viewpoint. Chapters 8 through 11 give you the opportunity to figure out what kinds and amounts of food your body requires for optimal fat burning and how to begin using *40-30-30 Fat-Burning Nutrition.* Chapter 12, Chapter 13, and the Appendix offer insight into restaurant eating, fast foods, supplements, a food shopping list, a chart to help you track your results, and a recommended reading list.

Remember

No program will work if you don't give it a fair chance. Simply follow the *40-30-30 Fat-Burning Nutrition* guidelines for at least two to six weeks and watch for results at the end of the second week. Don't worry about checking the scale every day. Instead, measure your results by how you look and feel, the way your clothes fit, improved strength and energy, and reduced hunger and carbohydrate cravings.

> 95 percent of all diets fail. Americans are eating less fat and more carbohydrates and are now <u>fatter than ever</u>!

Chapter 1

THE BIOSYN HUMAN PERFORMANCE CENTER

You may be wondering how we got involved in *40-30-30 Fat-Burning Nutrition* at a time when the high-carbohydrate, low-fat diet was all the rage. At one time, we were sales representatives for Tyson and Associates, a leading amino acid manufacturer. After years of training with Don Tyson, owner of Tyson and Associates, Inc., and his technical scientists on staff, we acquired quite an education in amino acids and we learned the vital importance of protein in the diet. We became technical advisors to doctors, nutritionists, health food store employers, trainers, and gym personnel in the area of dietary supplementation; Gene even became known as "The Amino Man."

Scientific Research

In 1991, we began working with Dr. Barry Sears, a scientist whose research exposed the negative effects of high-carbohydrate diets. His work promoted a diet consisting of 40 percent of the calories coming from carbohydrate, 30 percent from protein, and 30 percent from *good* fat. Since it suggested eating *higher* amounts of protein than the high-carbohydrate diets, we were interested.

We reviewed hundreds of amino acid profiles and we kept seeing amino acid deficiencies, even in our own. We were curious why Americans, who were supposed to be eating too much protein, were always showing up with amino acid deficiencies. Upon further research of the hormonal response of a high-carbohydrate diet, the 40-30-30 approach made a lot of sense.

We designed a diet for our specific requirements and followed it for one month. The results were outstanding:

> • Gene had been eating adequate protein and fat for his size, and simply had to reduce the high amount of carbohydrate in his diet. He quickly lost 12 pounds of pure body fat and gained 5 pounds of solid muscle.
>
> • Joyce was eating close to 75-80 percent carbohydrate and very little protein or fat. When she changed her diet to the *40-30-30* system, her body fat dropped from 23.7 percent to 17.3 percent and she added 4 pounds of lean muscle mass.

We had been taking plenty of high-quality vitamins, minerals, and amino acids, but we quickly realized that we had found the missing piece to the dietary puzzle: A balanced diet.

Testing 40-30-30 Ratio on Others

As a result of our fabulous personal success, we began testing the 40-30-30 ratio on others we knew who wanted to lose body fat. We worked with friends who needed to drop some excess body fat, bodybuilders who wanted to gain muscle and stay lean, as well as several aquaintances who were sick, using supplements, but still not experiencing good health. The results were unbelievable. Fat loss and sports performance were increased, and those who were sick and losing lean muscle mass were feeling better and gaining muscle.

At that point, things just fell into place. Early in 1992, we opened the BioSyn Human Performance Center in Kirkland, Washington, located next door to a very popular health club with over 30,000 members and just a few miles from the Seattle Seahawks training center.

Results, Results, Results!

We designed personalized 40-30-30 diets for our clients based on their size, body fat percentage, and activity level. We incorporated the use of a 40-30-30 meal replacement nutrition bar for the convenience of our clients when they couldn't prepare a well-balanced meal. We began working with hundreds of average individuals, as well as advanced professional athletes and their trainers. The center was an instant success for three reasons: One, the meals we recommended made sense and were easy to follow. Two, the 40-30-30 meal replacement nutrition bars tasted good and made following the program easier. Three, it worked. Women who had been training at the gym for months with no results from their high-carbohydrate diets were finally losing body fat and seeing muscle tone. The results were even better for men. They dropped fat and gained muscle and strength even faster than the women.

Women who had been training at the gym for months with no results from their high-carbohydrate diets were finally losing body fat and seeing muscle tone.

Then the media found out about us. A local television news station came to our center and videotaped us working with clients and testing body fat. The reporters interviewed our clients about their before and after experiences and they spoke with the trainer of the Seattle Seahawks and many of the football players themselves. We just gave a simple explanation as to what a 40-30-30 balanced diet is and why the high-carbohydrate diets were obviously not working.

People Started Talking

A few weeks later, the TV station ran a 2 1/2 minute spot on a very popular nightly local news show and it was like a dam had broken. Our phone began to ring at 7:23 that night and it didn't slow

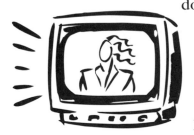

down for two weeks. We were getting thousands of phone calls an hour. The phone company told us their main circuits were overloaded. We were set up for voice mail and had to hire a Kelly girl just to retrieve messages for eight hours a day. Viewers from Washington, Oregon, and Canada had seen the show and were determined to find out more about the 40-30-30 program. It obviously hit a chord with thousands that the high-carbohydrate diet was keeping them fat and that the 40-30-30 ratio made perfect sense.

Doctors began turning to us for nutritional advice, because some of their patients using the 40-30-30 program were dropping body fat, reducing cholesterol and blood pressure, and raving about us and our program.

After only a few months, we began compiling the data on our clients. The results were astounding. The average women we worked with had a starting body fat percentage of 29 percent. For men, the figure was 20 percent. These figures were not quite as high as the average but, remember, many of our clients were already exercising. The women on our program lost about 1 1/2 pounds of pure fat per week, with no muscle loss. Many actually *added* lean muscle mass. The men lost closer to 2 pounds of fat per week and gained almost that much in muscle mass. In some cases, the scale didn't change much, but our clients' overall appearance did. Body fat testing was a much more accurate measure of their results than just hopping on a scale. Word of mouth was our best advertising.

> **The results were astounding. Women on our program lost about 1 ¹/₂ pounds of pure fat per week, with no muscle loss.**

Now, we want to tell the entire world that *40-30-30 Fat-Burning Nutrition* is the greatest discovery ever in nutrition. We hope this book changes *your* dietary habits and helps you keep burning fat forever

40-30-30
FAT-BURNING NUTRITION

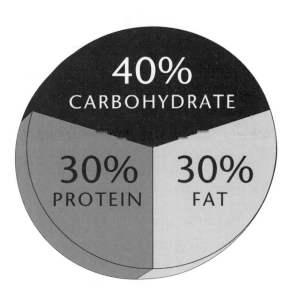

LOSING THE RIGHT KIND OF WEIGHT

40-30-30 Fat-Burning Nutrition is a dietary prescription of how to eat balanced meals to maximize the burning of stored body fat for energy through hormonal control. *Fat is the body's preferred source of energy, not carbohydrate.* We all have plenty of stored body fat to burn; doesn't it make sense to use that fat for energy instead of relying on carbohydrate? And when you start burning stored body fat for energy, not only will you have more energy and better concentration and mental focus, but you will look and feel great, since you are finally losing the right kind of weight—fat, not muscle.

> We all have plenty of stored body fat to burn; doesn't it make sense to use that fat for energy instead of relying on carbohydrates?

Controlling Fat-Burning Hormones

Unlike the high-carbohydrate or low-fat diets that are so popular today, *40-30-30 Fat-Burning Nutrition* uses a precise ratio of carbohydrate, protein, and fat eaten at every meal that can control the release of your body's powerful fat-burning hormones, so you can maximize the burning of stored body fat for energy.

We are convinced that *40-30-30 Fat-Burning Nutrition* is the greatest breakthrough ever in nutrition. We have seen it work successfully thousands of times for others. We know it can work for *you*.

UNDERSTANDING 40-30-30 FAT-BURNING NUTRITION

At the BioSyn Human Performance Center, our research confirmed that the ratio of carbohydrate, protein, and fat that produced the best results in weight loss, muscle gain, and fat burning was 40 percent carbohydrate, 30 percent protein, and 30 percent fat. To maximize the release of *your* fat-burning hormones, simply learn how to eat the correct 40-30-30 ratio of carbohydrate, protein, and fat at every meal. There really are no good or bad foods. The key is achieving the proper *balance* of the foods that you eat.

Chapter 8 provides complete meal guidelines to show you the exact amount of food and the correct balance of carbohydrate, protein, and fat that you should maintain. *40-30-30 Fat-Burning Nutrition* meals contain 40 percent of the calories from high-fiber and predominantly low-glycemic carbohydrate, with 30 percent high-quality protein, and 30 percent fat. *Another way to look at it is to have 1/3 more carbohydrate than protein (a 1.3 to 1 ratio), and one small serving of fat per meal.*

> *When you start burning stored body fat for energy…you will look and feel great since you are finally losing the right kind of weight —fat, not muscle.*

The Key to Unlocking Your Fat

A moderate amount of carbohydrate, protein, and a little fat helps keep blood sugar balanced. Fat slows down the digestion and absorption of the carbohydrate, providing a steady, ongoing supply of glucose which keeps the fat storage hormone insulin low. Protein in a meal stimulates the release of the fat-burning hormone, glucagon, thereby maximizing your ability to burn stored body fat for energy.

40% of Total Calories from Carbohydrate

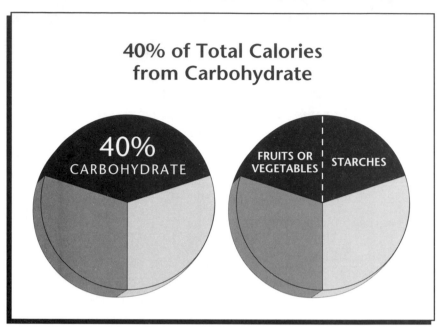

1/3 More Carbohydrate Than Protein
(1.3 to 1 Carbohydrate to Protein Ratio)

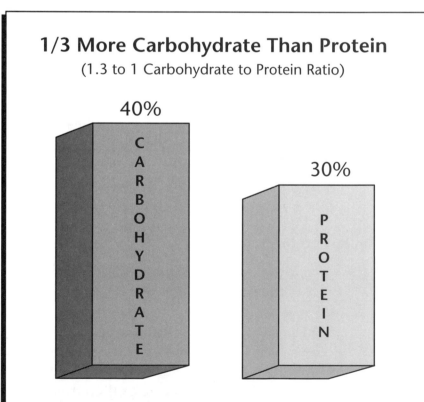

40 Percent Carbohydrate

There are three *macronutri- ents*—food sources needed by your body in large amounts—re- quired for proper nutrition. One of the three macronutrients is car- bohydrate. If you know what foods consist primarily of protein (beef, chicken, dairy, eggs, fish, pork, etc), and what foods consist primarily of fat (butter, oil, nuts, seeds, etc.), you are left with carbohydrate. Breads, fruits, juices, legumes, starches, vegetables, whole grains, and all sugary sweet foods consist primarily of carbohydrate.

When you eat high-carbohydrate foods, the body digests them and converts them into glucose (blood sugar) which enters the bloodstream to be burned as energy. Your body also converts glucose into glycogen which is stored in your muscles and liver. When small amounts of car- bohydrate are eaten in a meal, a small amount of glucose enters the blood- stream and is immediately used for energy.

> **Eat carbohydrates that are high in fiber, low in starch, and low in sugar.**

The problems begin when you eat a meal that is *too high* in carbohydrate (for example, a bagel and juice, a plate of pasta, or a sugary brownie). This is because too much glucose enters the blood- stream too rapidly. A high-carbohydrate meal stimu- lates a biochemical response that forces your body to burn glucose rather than stored body fat as its main source of fuel.

When you eat carbohydrates, the best advice is to eat carbohydrates that are high in fiber, low in starch, and low in sugar. Some of the best *40-30-30 Fat-Burning Nutrition* carbohydrate sources include:

Fruits	Apples, apricots, cherries, grapefruits, oranges, peaches, plums
Vegetables	Artichokes, asparagus, broccoli, cauliflower, green beans
Grains	Oatmeal, rye, wild rice
Legumes	Black beans, chick peas, kidney beans, lentils
Starches	Sweet potatoes, whole grain pasta, yams

* For a complete food list see Chapter 11 and the Glycemic Index in Chapter 4.

How Much Carbohydrate Do You Need?

In *40-30-30 Fat-Burning Nutrition,* we recommend that 40 percent of your total daily calories come from carbohydrate. Exactly how much carbohydrate you need can be calculated by first determining how much protein you need, then simply adding 1/3 more carbohydrate than protein (a 1.3 to 1 ratio of carbohydrate to protein) every time you eat.

40-30-30 Fat-Burning Nutrition uses balanced meals containing high-fiber carbohydrate. In Chapter 4, "The Glycemic Index," we explain why all carbohydrates are not created equal and why this is of importance to you. In Chapter 8, *"Putting It All Together,"* we show you the best type and amount of carbohydrate that you should have.

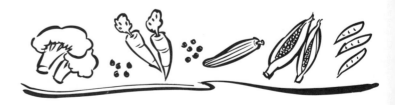

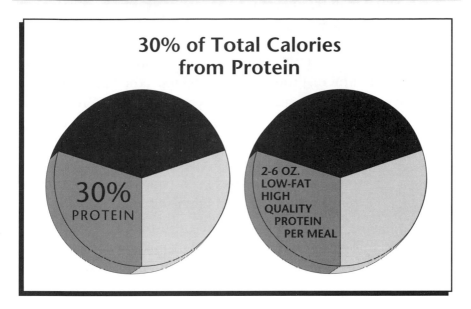

30% of Total Calories from Protein

30%
PROTEIN

2-6 OZ.
LOW-FAT
HIGH
QUALITY
PROTEIN
PER MEAL

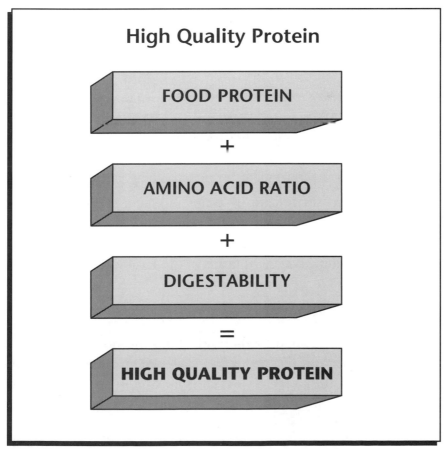

High Quality Protein

FOOD PROTEIN

+

AMINO ACID RATIO

+

DIGESTABILITY

=

HIGH QUALITY PROTEIN

30 Percent Protein

One of the most important macronutrients is protein. Protein is referred to as the "building blocks of life" because the body uses protein to rebuild and repair itself. More than half of your dry body weight consists of protein. This includes muscle, hair, skin, nails, blood, hormones, enzymes, brain neurotransmitters, and much more. Even your immune system requires protein to maintain itself.

When you eat high-protein foods such as chicken, eggs, fish, and so forth, the digestive process breaks down the protein chains into amino acids. Once the protein chains are digested into amino acids, they enter the bloodstream and are transformed into more than 50,000 new body proteins. Essential amino acids are the 10 amino acids that are found in food that the human body cannot make on its own.

> *It is vitally important that every time you eat, you supply your body with adequate amounts of quality protein containing sufficient ratios of the 10 essential amino acids.*

The body cannot store excess amino acids the way it can carbohydrate and fat. It is therefore vitally important that every time you eat, you supply your body with adequate amounts of quality protein containing sufficient ratios of the 10 essential amino acids.

The Right Amount of Protein in Your Diet

If your diet is lacking the proper amount of protein, or you are not digesting protein adequately, or the protein you eat is lacking in any of the 10 essential amino acids, your body's ability to make new body proteins slows down and you actually start to *break down* existing body protein (such as muscle) to supply the body with the amino acids that your food is lacking. When this protein breakdown process occurs, it is the *worst* possible thing that could happen. This is because you sacrifice muscle (your fat-burning machines) and your metabolism slows *way* down. As a result, your body actually burns *less* calories and fat. This is why you can lose muscle tone on high-carbohydrate diets that are too low in protein.

Protein is the *only* macronutrient that builds and maintains muscle. Muscle is also known as your lean body mass or LBM. Your LBM will ultimately determine how much stored body fat your body will burn. LBM is the magic bullet for increasing your metabolism; the more muscle you have, the faster your metabolism is, and the more stored body fat and calories you burn.

Adequate quality protein is the most critical component of *40-30-30 Fat-Burning Nutrition.* Based on your lean muscle mass, you require a specific amount of protein each day. Every meal or snack that you eat should contain a portion of your total protein requirements. Never skip eating your protein at breakfast or lunch so you can save it all up for dinner. If you do, your body will store fat instead of burning it.

> **Never skip eating your protein at breakfast or lunch....if you do, your body will store fat instead of burning it.**

In Chapter 8 *"Putting It All Together,"* you will find specific diet plans for different size individuals. By choosing the right plan, you will be getting adequate protein, carbohydrate, and fat at each meal throughout the day.

Some of the best *40-30-30 Fat-Burning Nutrition* sources of high-quality protein foods that are low in fat, low in fiber, and easy to digest include:

- Cottage cheese (low-fat)
- Eggs and egg whites
- Fish
- Lean meats
- Low-fat tofu and tempeh
- Skinless turkey and chicken
- Whey protein powder

* For a complete food list see Chapter 11.

How Much Protein Do You Need?

In *40-30-30 Fat-Burning Nutrition* we recommend that 30 percent of your total daily calories come from protein. Exactly how much protein you need is determined by your size and activity level. The bigger you are and more activity that you undertake, the more protein you need to keep your fat-burning machines (muscles) working as efficiently as possible. In general, you need anywhere from .5 to 1 gram of protein per one pound of body weight per day.

40-30-30 Fat-Burning Nutrition uses balanced meals containing high-quality protein. In Chapter 8, *"Putting It All Together,"* we will show you the best low-fat protein foods and the amounts that you should have each day.

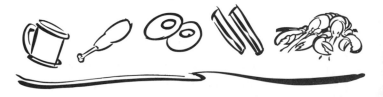

40-30-30 Fat-Burning Nutrition uses balanced meals containing "good" fat. In Chapter 8, *"Putting It All Together,"* we show you the best fat sources and the amounts that you should have each day.

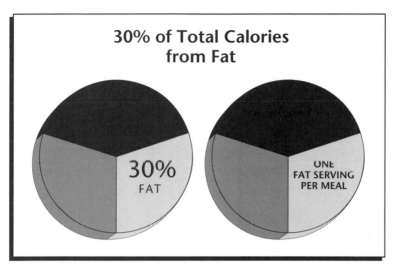

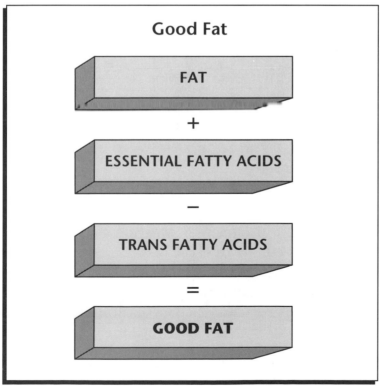

30 Percent Fat

Fat is certainly the most misunderstood of the three macronutrients. Contrary to what we have been told, not all fat is "bad." We all *need* fat in our diets to help burn *stored* body fat. Just like carbohydrate and protein, fat is beneficial in appropriate quantities, but it is harmful to ingest either too much or too little of it. Eating the right kind and amount of fat is essential for good health and proper fat metabolism. Dietary fat provides us an important source of essential fatty acids, slows the digestive process (which helps us feel satisfied after meals), and plays a critical role in the body's hormonal response to food.

Fat in the diet provides you with:
- Energy
- The release of CCK, a hormone that signals the brain that you're full and to stop eating
- Fat-soluble compounds for proper metabolism of fat-soluble vitamins
- Omega 3 and Omega 6 fatty acids, necessary for fat metabolism and production of eicosanoids
- A control mechanism to slow the rate of carbohydrate into the bloodstream and reduce the rate of insulin secretion

Contrary to what the so-called experts say, stored body fat is the body's preferred source of energy, not carbohydrate. In fact, most of us have enough energy stored as body fat to run several marathons back-to-back. Doesn't it makes sense to burn stored body fat for energy instead of carbohydrate?

General guidelines recommend that total fat intake should not exceed 30 percent of your daily total calories. Ideally, you should eat all three varieties of fat in equal proportions: 10 percent saturated, 10 percent unsaturated, and 10 percent monounsaturated. Saturated fats are found predominately in animal meats, unsaturated fats in vegetable oils, and monounsaturated fats primarily in vegetables, avocados, canola oil, and olives.

The "good" fats are unprocessed and occur naturally in foods. The "bad" fats are called *trans* fats, since they contain trans fatty acids, and are found in hydrogenated oils. Hydrogenated oils are high in almost all processed foods and margarine, and should be kept to a minimum or avoided altogether.

Some of the best *40-30-30 Fat-Burning Nutrition* sources of "good" fats that are naturally occurring and unprocessed are:

- Avocados
- Cold water fish (salmon, mackerel, tuna, herring, crab, etc.)
- Raw nuts, nut butters, and seeds
- Safflower-based mayonnaise
- Vegetable oils (olive oil, safflower, sesame, sunflower)

* For a complete food list see Chapter 11.

How Much Fat Do You Need?

In *40-30-30 Fat-Burning Nutrition* we recommend that 30 percent of your daily total calories come from fat. You need the same amount of calories from fat as you do from protein, but because fat contains nine calories per gram and protein has only four, your fat grams will be less than half your protein grams.

Fat: The Building Block for Your Body's Super Hormones—Eicosanoids

Not only is the fat in your diet important to burn stored body fat and slow digestion, but it is also the macronutrient precursor for the class of hormones known as eicosanoids. Originally discovered in the 1930s, eicosanoids can be thought of as the master control panel for all of the body's functions. In the 1970s and 1980s, scientists extensively explored the eicosanoid family of hormones and its relationship to disease. Today, researchers are redefining wellness in terms of the balance of "good" and "bad" eicosanoids.

It is not so important to understand the role of all of these substances, but more so the powerful effects that they have on the human body. Just as with all other hormones, they have directly opposite physiological actions in the body—in simpler terms, "good" *and* "bad" effects. Your ultimate goal is to strive for your body to produce more "good" eicosanoids and less "bad," resulting in the right balance for optimal health.

> **Stored body fat is the body's preferred source of energy, not carbohydrates....Most of us have enough energy stored as body fat to run several marathons back-to-back.**

So how can you control the production of good and bad eicosanoids? By the foods you eat. Dietary fat provides us with essential fatty acids (Omega 3 and Omega 6) that are the macronutrient building blocks for eicosanoid production. The balance of carbohydrate and protein in a meal controls the insulin-to-glucagon ratio, which determines "bad" or "good" eicosanoid production.

Understanding the Dietary Hormonal Connection to Burning Fat

Chapter 3

If your diet is too high in carbohydrates, your body will produce too much insulin. This will invariably result in the production of bad eicosanoids. But if every meal you eat is balanced with a 40-30-30 ratio of carbohydrate, protein, and fat (decreasing the production of insulin and increasing the production of glucagon), you will have better control over the hormonal response of foods—thus ensuring the production of ample amounts of good eicosanoids.

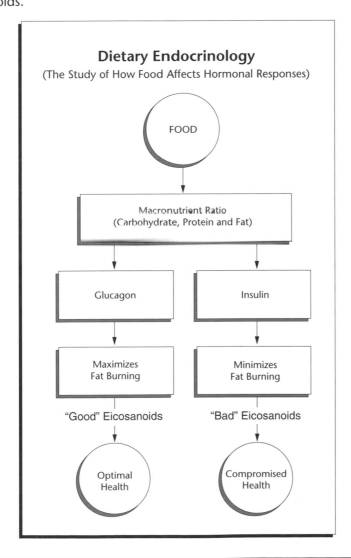

Dietary Endocrinology
(The Study of How Food Affects Hormonal Responses)

FOOD

Macronutrient Ratio
(Carbohydrate, Protein and Fat)

| Glucagon | Insulin |

| Maximizes Fat Burning | Minimizes Fat Burning |

"Good" Eicosanoids | "Bad" Eicosanoids

Optimal Health | Compromised Health

THE POWER OF HORMONES

Hormones regulate virtually everything your body does. Therefore, it's not hard to understand that hormones can be very powerful in determining whether you burn fat or store it. It sounds so easy, and it is. Simply eat the meals that stimulate the fat-burning hormone and don't eat the meals that stimulate the fat storage hormone.

Although it's easy, most people have been doing it all wrong. If your diet has been loaded with carbohydrate, especially high-glycemic carbohydrate, or is too low in protein and fat, you have been unknowingly stimulating the fat-storing hormone insulin and suppressing the fat-burning hormone glucagon. Let's see how these powerful hormones work.

> **Hormones can be very powerful in determining whether you burn or store fat. Simply eat the right meals that stimulate fat-burning hormones.**

Understanding the Dietary Hormones

To truly understand the benefits of *40-30-30 Fat-Burning Nutrition*, it is necessary to learn about how the balance of carbohydrate, protein, and fat in the food you eat affects the hormones that your body produces to store and burn fat.

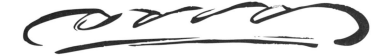

INSULIN—THE FAT STORAGE HORMONE

Insulin can be viewed as your body's fat storage hormone. Insulin is a hormone that is secreted by the pancreas in response to elevated blood sugar (glucose) levels—primarily from ingesting excessive carbohydrate in a meal. One of insulin's big jobs in the human body is to decrease blood glucose levels when they get too high.

It is important that an individual's blood sugar level does not rise too high or too quickly because, if it does, the body reacts by alerting the pancreas. The pancreas then detects the excess glucose and secretes the hormonal messenger, insulin, to correct it. Increased levels of insulin force your body to burn glucose for energy, and store any excess away as glycogen or fat.

Elevated Insulin Levels

As a result of this process, elevated insulin levels prevent your body from burning stored body fat for energy. This is because insulin converts excess blood glucose into glycogen, removes it from the bloodstream, and stores it in your liver and muscles. Unfortunately, the excess glucose that your body cannot store as glycogen will be converted to *new* fat and stored in your adipose tissue—your butt, hips, back, and so forth.

If blood sugar levels rise too high or too quickly your body is forced to burn glucose for energy and store any excess glucose away as glycogen or fat.

Remember, this entire response is primarily the result of eating too much carbohydrate and not enough protein and fat as a part of your meal.

One more thing: raised insulin levels can also stimulate "bad" eicosanoid production. This causes blood vessels to get smaller or constrict (vasoconstriction). When blood vessels constrict, there is less oxygen available in your body to burn fat. To burn fat efficiently, oxygen must be present—and lots of it. This is why aerobic exercise works best to burn fat.

Here are the main reasons why elevated insulin levels can hamper your attempts to burn body fat:

- Your body is forced to burn carbohydrate for energy instead of stored fat.
- The release and utilization of stored body fat for energy is inhibited.
- Your body converts and stores excess glucose as body fat.
- The production of "bad" eicosanoids cause vasoconstriction which decreases the amount of oxygen available to burn body fat.

You *cannot* maximize fat burning with elevated levels of insulin. It's that simple. Even if you exercise like crazy, elevated insulin levels will *not* maximize fat burning. Even worse, elevated insulin levels will stimulate your body to *store* fat.

Elevated insulin levels can be caused by any of these three key dietary factors:

- Eating too much carbohydrate in a meal or snack.
- Eating too large of a meal.
- Not eating *enough* protein and fat in a meal or snack.

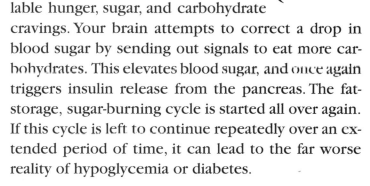

Besides not burning fat, elevated insulin levels can cause blood sugar concentrations to drop too low, leaving you to suffer the effects of low blood sugar. These effects include loss of concentration; mood swings; fatigue; low energy; and uncontrollable hunger, sugar, and carbohydrate cravings. Your brain attempts to correct a drop in blood sugar by sending out signals to eat more carbohydrates. This elevates blood sugar, and once again triggers insulin release from the pancreas. The fat-storage, sugar-burning cycle is started all over again. If this cycle is left to continue repeatedly over an extended period of time, it can lead to the far worse reality of hypoglycemia or diabetes.

If high-carbohydrate diets increase blood sugar too much, resulting in elevated insulin levels, why not just go on a low-carbohydrate diet? The answer is right between your ears. It's your brain.

The human brain is a glucose hog and it requires a constant supply of glucose for fuel. When blood sugar spikes up from eating too much carbohydrate, insulin is released to lower it. If blood sugar drops too low, the brain calls out for more. The glucose-starved brain then sends out signals of low

Elevated insulin levels can cause ...loss of concentration, mood swings, fatigue, low energy, and uncontrollable hunger.

blood sugar (hypoglycemia), which can initiate loss of concentration, mood swings, fatigue, low energy, and out-of-control hunger and carbohydrate cravings.

On the other hand, restricting carbohydrates from your diet creates its own set of problems. Remember, your brain needs glucose. When your diet does not supply adequate carbohydrates, your body quickly uses up its available glucose and glycogen stores. The body and brain next turn to fat and muscle mass to supply energy—producing the abnormal metabolic state called ketosis. Ketosis alters the enzymes in fat cells. This results in abnormal fat breakdown, causing fat cells to react like fat *magnets*. When normal eating patterns return, fat accumulates in your body faster than ever.

> *95 percent of all of the low-carbohydrate diets and high-protein liquid diets fail and their users gain back any weight they may have lost—and usually more.*

Ketosis also causes muscle mass to be sacrificed and broken back down into amino acids to be converted directly into glucose for the brain. It becomes easy to see why 95 percent of all of the low-carbohydrate diets and high-protein liquid diets fail and their users gain back any weight they may have lost—and usually more.

Protein Sparing Effect

Finally, carbohydrate also has what is known as a protein sparing effect. When you eat the right balance of carbohydrate, protein, and fat in a meal, the carbohydrate that you ingest provides adequate glucose for your body's needs, eliminating the necessity of breaking down and metabolizing your muscle tissue into glucose. This preserves lean muscle mass and maximizes fat burning. When your diet is properly balanced, the hormonal response created allows the muscles to access and burn stored body fat for energy, sparing glucose for the brain. When insulin and glucagon maintain a harmonious balance, the body runs efficiently and at peak performance.

GLUCAGON—THE FAT MOBILIZATION HORMONE

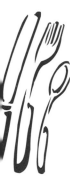

Glucagon works in a completely opposite way from insulin and is therefore considered the fat-*burning* hormone. Glucagon is stimulated by the pancreas, primarily in response to the presence of adequate amounts of protein in the diet. Glucagon's primary job is to maintain stable blood sugar levels in your body. It does this by mobilizing stored body fat so it can be burned for energy.

> Stimulating insulin release by eating excessive carbohydrate lowers the level of glucagon. This is precisely the wrong homonal response if you want to burn body fat.

Stimulating the Release of Glucagon—The Right Way

By eating protein in a meal, along with the right balance of carbohydrate and fat, you can stabilize blood sugar concentrations and stimulate the release of glucagon. Glucagon is like a magic bullet for burning fat because it mobilizes the release of stored body fat from the adipose tissue directly into the bloodstream, allowing your muscle cells to burn fat (their preferred source of fuel) instead of blood sugar for energy.

Glucagon also stimulates "good" eicosanoid production by your body. This causes your blood vessels to get larger, or dilate (vasodilation). When blood vessels dilate, you have *more* oxygen available to burn fat. With more oxygen available, you stay in aerobic metabolism longer, thereby maximizing your body's ability to burn fat.

Elevated glucagon levels enable the body to burn stored body fat by:

- Enabling the body to burn stored body fat for energy instead of glucose.
- Stimulating the release of stored body fat so it can be burned for energy.
- Mobilizing the release of stored liver and muscle glycogen to maintain stable blood sugar levels.
- Stimulating vasodilation which increases the amount of oxygen available to burn fat.

It is important to remember that insulin and glucagon are complete opposites, but paired hormones. This means that when the level of insulin is elevated, the level of glucagon is lowered. Conversely, when the level of insulin is lowered, the level of glucagon is elevated. So, when you stimulate insulin release by eating excessive carbohydrate in a meal, you are also lowering the level of your fat-burning hormone glucagon at the same time. This is precisely the *wrong* hormonal response if you want to burn body fat.

However, with 40-30-30 *Fat-Burning Nutrition*, you can stabilize blood sugar levels and maintain a favorable balance of insulin to glucagon. This allows your body to mobilize and access stored body fat as your primary source of fuel, while sparing the glucose that you need for your brain.

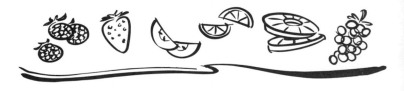

Elevated levels of glucagon can be caused by three key dietary factors:

- Eating adequate amounts of protein in a meal or snack.
- Controlling the amount and type of carbohydrate in a meal or snack.
- Including a small amount of "good" fat in a meal or snack.

When blood sugar is stable, the level of glucagon is elevated, allowing the body to access and burn stored body fat for energy. If you learn how to stabilize blood sugar levels by your food choices and maintain the favorable balance of insulin to glucagon, you can maximize fat burning 24 hours a day, *every* day—even while you sleep or while you are reading this book.

THE HORMONAL POWER OF EXERCISE

40-30-30 Fat-Burning Nutrition can set your body up hormonally to burn fat faster so you can get the most from your exercise.

So how does exercise reduce body fat? It burns calories and increases the metabolic rate, but even more powerful are the *hormonal* benefits of exercise. High-intensity aerobic exercise reduces insulin and increases glucagon, the fat mobilization hormone. In addition, anaerobic exercise (strength training), will stimulate the body to release HGH (human growth hormone), the body's most *powerful* fat-burning hormone. HGH is doubly powerful because it burns fat as well as playing a crucial role in building and repairing muscle. Aerobic exercise coupled with anaerobic exercise lowers body fat and increases lean muscle mass.

MAXIMIZING YOUR PERFORMANCE

When you load up on carbohydrate before, during, or right after exercise, you are doing everything possible to inhibit glucagon and HGH release by stimulating insulin and forcing your body to burn carbohydrate instead of stored body fat. This completely negates the hormonal benefits of exercise. Using *40-30-30 Fat-Burning Nutrition* is like priming the fat-burning hormone pump. It stabilizes blood sugar levels, keeps insulin low, and elevates the fat-burning hormones, glucagon and HGH.

Burning Fat Instead of Carbohydrate

Don't forget: you get over twice as much energy from burning stored body fat than you do from burning sugars. One gram of fat will provide you with nine calories or units of energy, while one gram of carbohydrate provides only four. So, not only do you have a lot of energy stored as body fat but, when you start burning stored body fat, you get an explosion of energy that goes far beyond what you will ever get from burning carbohydrate.

And glucagon promotes vasodilation, which widens blood vessels so more oxygen and nutrients can get to your muscles and more lactic acid can get out. This increases performance and recovery while keeping

> You get over twice as much energy from burning stored body fat than you do from burning sugars.

you in aerobic metabolism longer. Stabilizing blood sugar levels keeps your brain performing at peak levels by keeping adequate amounts of glucose available and eliminating brain fatigue.

So, no matter what sport or activity you do, *40-30-30 Fat-Burning Nutrition* can help maximize your performance physically and mentally, and improve recovery. As you prepare to exercise, remember that the hormonal response you create during periods of exertion is controlled by the ratio of carbohydrate, protein, and fat in the last meal that you ate before your workout.

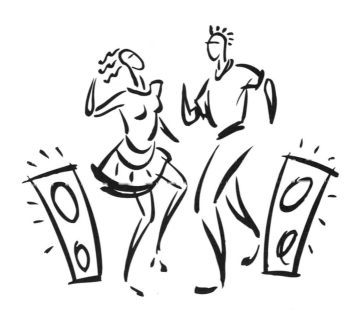

Maximizing Your Fat-Burning Hormones

High Carbohydrate Diets

HIGH BLOOD SUGAR

(Hyperglycemia)

Stimulates Fat Storage Hormone—Insulin

*Inhibits Fat Burning • Forces Sugar Burning
Severe Blood Sugar Swings • Loss of Muscle Tone and Shape
Energy and Endurance Swings • Slower Metabolism
Poor Mental Focus and Concentration • Mood Swings
Water Retention*

40-30-30 Fat-Burning Nutrition

BALANCED BLOOD SUGAR

Stimulates Your Fat-Burning Hormones

*Maximize Fat Burning • Balanced Blood Sugar
Maintain Muscle Tone and Shape • Increased Energy, Strength
and Endurance • Faster Metabolism • Better Mental Focus
and Concentration • Stable Moods*

Low Carbohydrate Diets

LOW BLOOD SUGAR

(Hypoglycemia)

Stimulates Ketosis, Causes Muscle Loss and Rapid Weight Regain

*Causes Ketosis • Low Blood Sugar (Hypoglycemia)
Loss of Muscle Tone and Shape • Low Energy and Endurance
Slow Metabolism • Lack of Mental Focus and Concentration
Poor Moods • Causes Ketosis and Bad Breath*

NOT ALL CARBOHYDRATES ARE CREATED EQUAL

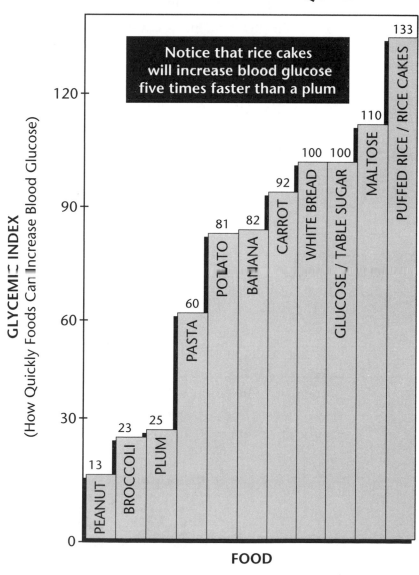

GLYCEMIC INDEX
(How Quickly Foods Can Increase Blood Glucose)

Notice that rice cakes will increase blood glucose five times faster than a plum

Food	Value
PEANUT	13
BROCCOLI	23
PLUM	25
PASTA	60
POTATO	81
BANANA	82
CARROT	92
WHITE BREAD	100
GLUCOSE / TABLE SUGAR	100
MALTOSE	110
PUFFED RICE / RICE CAKES	133

FOOD

NOT ALL CARBOHYDRATES ARE CREATED EQUAL

Most people have the impression that simple carbohydrates produce a major surge in blood glucose (sugar), whereas complex carbohydrates produce a flatter curve. We now know that this is not true. The effects of different foods on blood glucose depend on many factors. These effects are summarized by the glycemic index.

The glycemic index is a system that rates how quickly certain foods increase blood sugar levels and how quickly the body responds by bringing levels back to normal. The index was originally developed for diabetics. All foods were originally compared to pure glucose which is rated at 100. The higher the glycemic index number, the faster it raises blood sugar. The lower the glycemic index number, the slower the blood sugar will rise. The glycemic index of the food depends on the type of sugar in the carbohydrate, the amount of fiber in the food (the most important aspect), the amount of protein and fat in the food, and the method of cooking or processing of the food.

The glycemic index listed is easy to use, although not all foods have been rated. If you are interested in a food not listed, in general, the more fiber, protein, or fat in a food, the lower its glycemic index. Foods that are highly processed or high in refined sugars or flours are typically high-glycemic.

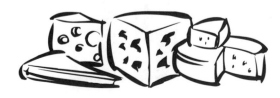

GLYCEMIC INDEX

FOODS	GLYCEMIC INDEX#

CEREALS

All Bran	74
Cornflakes	121
Muesli	96
Oat Bran	85
Oatmeal (instant)	89
Oatmeal (slow cooked)	49
Puffed Rice	132
Puffed Wheat	110
Shredded Wheat	97

COOKIES

Fat-Free Cookies	100+
Oatmeal	78
Shortbread	88
Water Biscuits	100

DAIRY

Custard	59
Ice Cream (full-fat)	69
Ice Cream (fat-free)	90+
Milk (skim)	46
Milk (whole)	44
Yogurt (plain, full-fat)	52
Yogurt (w/ fruit and sugar)	90+
Yogurt (frozen, fat-free)	90+
Yogurt (w/ fruit, artificial sugar)	63

FRUITS

Apple	49
Apple Juice (unfiltered)	55
Apple Sauce	52
Apricot	73
Banana	82
Cherries	23
Dates	95
Grapefruit	26
Grapes	45
Mango	78
Orange	59
Orange Juice	71
Papaya	75

FOODS	GLYCEMIC INDEX#

Peach	25
Pear	34
Plum	25
Prunes	52
Raisins	93

GRAINS

Barley (pearl)	36
Barley (rolled)	65
Bread (white)	100
Bread (wheat)	100
French Baguette	131
Puffed Crisp Bread	112
Buckwheat	78
Bulgur	65
Millet	81
Macaroni (boiled 5 min.)	66
Rice (brown or white)	81
Instant Rice (boiled 1 min.)	65
Instant Rice (boiled 6 min.)	121
Polished Rice (boiled 5 min.)	58
Polished Rice (boiled 10-25 min.)	83
Parboiled Rice (boiled 5 min.)	54
Parboiled Rice (boiled 15 min.)	68
Rye Bread (pumpernickel)	68
Rye Crisp Crackers	45
Rye Kernels	47
Rye Wholemeal	89
Spaghetti (brown, boiled 15 min.)	61
Spaghetti (white, boiled 15 min.)	67
Spaghetti (white, boiled 5 min.)	45
Pasta (protein enriched)	38
Wholemeal	100
White Flour	100
Wheat Kernels (pressure cooked)	63
Wheat Kernels (quick cooking)	75

NUTS

(Because of the high fat and protein content, all varieties of nuts have a very low-glycemic rating).

Almonds	15
Peanuts	15
Walnuts	15

GLYCEMIC INDEX

FOODS	GLYCEMIC INDEX#
SNACK FOODS	
Corn Chips	99
Popcorn	133
Potato Chips	77
Rice Cakes	132
Rice Cakes (apple-cinnamon flavored)	132+
SUGARS	
Fructose	26
Glucose	100
Honey	126
Lactose	57
Maltose	150
Sucrose	83
VEGETABLES AND LEGUMES	
(Almost all vegetables and legumes have a low- to very low-glycemic index rating).	
Artichoke (cooked)	25
Asparagus	22
Baked Beans	70
Beets	68
Black-Eyed Peas	53
Broccoli (raw)	23
Brussels Sprouts (raw)	23

FOODS	GLYCEMIC INDEX#
Carrots	92
Cauliflower (raw)	21
Chickpeas (dried)	47
Chickpeas (canned)	60
Corn (sweet)	76
Garbonzo beans	64
Kidney Beans (canned)	71
Kidney Beans (dried)	43
Lentils (green, dried)	36
Lentils (green, canned)	74
Lentils, (red, dried)	38
Lima Beans	46
Parsnips	96
Peas (green, dried)	50
Peas (frozen)	65
Pinto Beans (canned)	64
Pinto Beans (dried)	60
Potato (instant mashed)	120
Potato (mashed)	117
Potato (new, white, boiled)	80
Potato (new, red, boiled)	70
Potato (Russet, baked)	116
Soy Beans (canned)	22
Soy Beans (dried)	20
Sweet Potato	70
White Beans (dried)	54
Yam	74

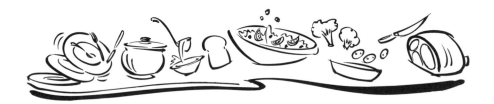

In general, the more fiber, protein, or fat in a food,
the lower its glycemic index. Foods that are highly
processed or high in refined sugars or flours
are typically high-glycemic.

WHY MOST CARBOHYDRATE DIETS FAIL

By reviewing the glycemic index, it is interesting to note that many diets encourage popcorn, rice cakes, potatoes, and carrots as acceptable snacks—all very high-glycemic foods. When eaten alone, high-glycemic foods produce a major surge in blood glucose and elevate insulin. This is why most high-carbohydrate diets fail and can actually get you fatter. Also, some processed complex carbohydrate foods elevate blood sugar 1/3 faster than pure sugar (glucose) when eaten alone.

A food's glycemic effect differs when it is eaten alone or as part of a balanced meal. When you combine high-glycemic carbohydrate, like potatoes and carrots, with protein and fat, like a chicken breast, to create a balanced meal, it will result in a much *lower* overall glycemic effect.

Using the glycemic index can be *very* helpful when choosing what carbohydrates to eat to maximize the fat burning process. Many people see faster fat loss using low- or medium-glycemic rated carbohydrates. The FBN Fat-Flush Meals in Chapter 8 use a combination of only low- and medium-glycemic index carbohydrates rated at 60 or less. An added benefit of lower-glycemic carbohydrates is that they are usually the most nutritious—loaded with vitamins, minerals, and fiber.

Listed on the next page are examples of *40-30-30 Fat-Burning Nutrition* meals using a variety of differently glycemic-rated carbohydrates.

**40-30-30 Fat-Burning Nutrition
Using Low-Glycemic Carbohydrates**

    1/2 c. 2% cottage cheese

    1 c. sliced peaches *(low-glycemic rating)*

    1 t. almonds

**40-30-30 Fat-Burning Nutrition
Using Medium-Glycemic Carbohydrates**

    1/2 c. 2% cottage cheese

    1 medium sliced apple with skin *(medium-glycemic rating)*

    1 t. almonds

**40-30-30 Fat-Burning Nutrition
Using High-Glycemic Carbohydrates**

    1/2 c. 2% cottage cheese

    1 banana, small *(high-glycemic rating)*

    1 t. almonds

**40-30-30 Fat-Burning Nutrition
Using Very High-Glycemic Carbohydrates**

    1/2 c. 2% cottage cheese

    3 rice cakes, plain or flavored *(very high-glycemic rating)*

    1 t. almonds

All of these meals are well balanced using the 40-30-30 ratio. However, the two meals containing the low- and medium-glycemic rated carbohydrate sources will produce a much lower blood sugar response than the high- or very high-glycemic rated carbohydrate sources.

40-30-30 Fat-Burning Nutrition Compared with Other Diets

Chapter 5

WHY DON'T DIETS WORK?

There are many diets being promoted to help burn fat or lose weight. Statistics show, however, that 95 percent of all diets fail to produce long-term success. So why don't diets work? The problem is that they fail to take into consideration the hormonal consequences of the foods they recommend. Listed below are a few of the most common diet approaches and the main problems associated with them.

High-Carbohydrate Diets

Today's most popular high-carbohydrate diets promote eating high amounts of carbohydrate, with low amounts of fat and protein.

The Problem—Stimulating the Fat-Storage Hormone, Insulin

Since high-carbohydrate diets are not balanced, they can cause blood sugar imbalances and trigger constant hunger with fatigue and mood swings. This leads to a failure to produce long-term success rates. Inadequate protein intake causes a loss of lean muscle mass and low fat intake contributes to hunger and potential fatty acid deficiencies. High amounts of carbohydrate, without the control factors of adequate protein and fat, elevate blood sugar levels. This stimulates the release of insulin. Elevated insulin levels force the body to burn sugars for energy, prevent the body from releasing and using its stored body fat for energy, and convert excess glucose into body fat.

Liquid Diets

Liquid diets promote low-calorie shakes as meal replacements which are high in protein, but very low in calories, carbohydrate, and fat. They should always be medically supervised.

The Problem—Promoting Ketosis and Muscle Loss

Liquid diets can produce rapid weight loss, but 90 percent of the users regain all of their weight *and more* when they begin to eat regular food again. Liquid diets cause ketosis which alters the enzymes in fat cells so they seek out and store fat like magnets. The excessively high amount of protein also stimulates insulin which triggers hunger, causes blood sugar fluctuations, and promotes muscle loss. And if that's not bad enough, ketosis inhibits the release of glucagon, the fat-burning hormone.

High-Protein, High-Fat, Low-Carbohydrate Diets

These diets promote high protein and high fat in meals, keeping carbohydrate to a bare minimum.

The Problem—Promoting Ketosis and Muscle Loss

This type of diet supplies plenty of calories, but not enough carbohydrate for glucose production. This results in brain fatigue, mood swings, and poor concentration. High-protein, high-fat, low-carbohydrate diets contain too much fat, which promotes a sluggish feeling. Excessive saturated fat in the diet can lead to high cholesterol, heart disease, and cancer. In addition, ketogenic diets cause bad breath and inhibit the release of glucagon, since too many calories in a meal can stimulate insulin.

The ultimate reason the previous diets fail is the negative hormonal response they create.

40-30-30 FAT-BURNING NUTRITION

First of all, *40-30-30 Fat-Burning Nutrition* is not a *diet* but a *dietary prescription* that trains your body to maximize fat burning through hormonal response. It promotes a balanced approach to nutrition by using meals containing 40 percent of the calories from predominately low-glycemic, high-fiber carbohydrate, 30 percent from low-fat, high-quality and easy-to-digest protein, and 30 percent from high-quality "good" fat.

The Solution—Promoting the Fat-Burning Hormone Glucagon

By eating moderate amounts of carbohydrate, protein, and fat at each meal, blood sugar levels remain stable and a favorable glucagon-to-insulin ratio is obtained.

Your body has better access to stored body fat for energy without sacrificing lean muscle mass.

 There's no big secret to burning fat. It's simply a matter of balance.

Listed on the next page is an example of a typical high-carbohydrate breakfast, and an example of a *40-30-30 Fat-Burning Nutrition* breakfast. Notice the difference between the meals and decide for yourself which one would be most likely to increase insulin or increase glucagon.

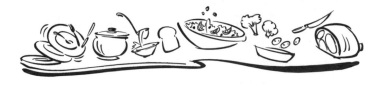

SAMPLE BREAKFASTS

High-Carbohydrate Diet	**40-30-30 Fat-Burning Nutrition**
2.5 oz. raisin bagel	2.5 oz. bagel
1 banana	1.5 oz. cream cheese
8 oz. orange juice	3 oz. turkey breast, sliced
coffee or tea	1/2 orange
	coffee or tea

TOTALS	CALORIES	CARB.	PROTEIN	FAT	RATIO CARB/PROT
High-Carb. Diet	438	96 g	9 g	2 g	10 to 1
40-30-30 FBN	416	49 g	37 g	16 g	1.3 to 1

The high-carbohydrate diet has a greater than 10 to 1 ratio of carbohydrate to protein. It consists primarily of high-glycemic carbohydrates and is very low in quality protein. This is a hormonal *nightmare* if your goal is to burn fat and lose the right kind of weight—body fat. Ultimately, the high-carbohydrate, low-protein, and very low-fat diet can slow your metabolism and cause you to burn even *less* fat.

The *40-30-30 Fat-Burning Nutrition* breakfast contains the proper 40-30-30 ratio. It has a 1.3 to 1 ratio of carbohydrate to protein (or 1/3 more carbohydrate than protein), the dietary prescription to stimulating your fat burning hormones and losing the right kind of weight—fat! Both high- and low-glycemic carbohydrate are combined with protein and fat in the meal to help keep blood sugar levels balanced.

> The high-carbohydrate diet is a hormonal nightmare if your goal is to burn fat and lose the right kind of weight—body fat.

The protein and small amount of fat slows carbohydrate digestion and absorption, keeping you full for 4-6 hours. It also supplies essential fatty acids needed for proper hormone production. High-quality protein will support body proteins, maintain muscle tone and shape, and keep your metabolism high.

Moderate amounts of protein in the meal also stimulate the release of the fat-burning hormone, glucagon, so you maximize your body's ability to burn stored body fat for energy.

WHAT ABOUT DIET PILLS?

There are many diet pills being sold today. Stimulants, fat burners, and herbal products are readily available. The underlying message we want to convey is that there are *no* magic pills or potions. You still have to eat food that will stimulate either a *positive* or *negative* fat-burning hormonal response. The most *powerful* fat burner on the planet today is simply the food we put in our mouth.

WHAT ABOUT JUICING?

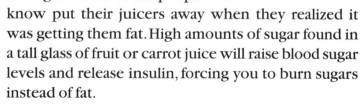

Fruit and some vegetable juice is typically very high in carbohydrates and natural sugars. Most of the people we know put their juicers away when they realized it was getting them fat. High amounts of sugar found in a tall glass of fruit or carrot juice will raise blood sugar levels and release insulin, forcing you to burn sugars instead of fat.

Juicing can be used with *40-30-30 Fat-Burning Nutrition*, but only if you use *small* amounts of the high-sugar fruits and vegetables. For best results, have one ounce of juice from high-sugar containing sweet fruits and vegetables and the rest from green vegetables. Our suggestion is to eat your fruits and vegetables whole with the fiber in them as part of a balanced meal and keep juicing to a minimum.

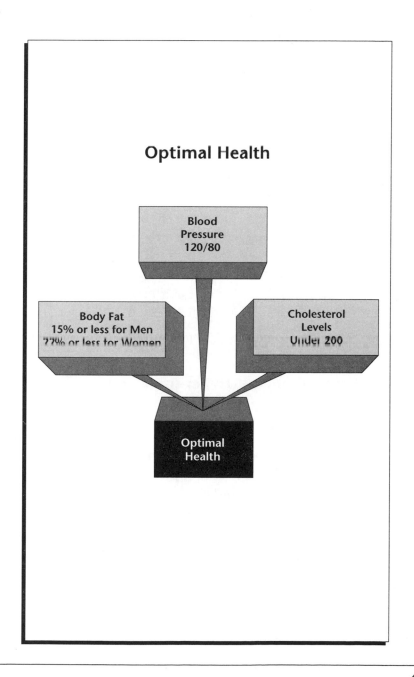

OTHER BENEFITS OF 40-30-30 FAT-BURNING NUTRITION

40-30-30 Fat-Burning Nutrition is *not* just for losing body fat. While burning fat may be your primary motivation for using *40-30-30 Fat-Burning Nutrition*, consider some of these other health benefits:

Mental Performance

Your brain needs glucose (blood sugar) for energy. When you eat too much carbohydrate, blood sugar rises too fast, stimulating the release of insulin to lower it. In many cases, blood sugar then drops too low. This short circuits the brain's supply of energy causing it to tune out (brain bonk). *40-30-30 Fat-Burning Nutrition* can help keep blood sugar balanced and improve your overall mental focus and concentration.

> 40-30-30 Fat-Burning Nutrition can help keep blood sugar balanced and improve your overall mental focus and concentration.

Type II Diabetes (Hyperinsulinemia)

Type II diabetes is also known as hyperinsulinemia (high levels of insulin). It is the predominant type of diabetes and is characterized by cells becoming less receptive to insulin. When this happens, more and more insulin is needed to reduce high blood glucose levels. *40-30-30 Fat-Burning Nutrition* is designed to keep blood glucose from rising too high, thereby helping to control the body's production of insulin. This helps to reduce the risk of developing type II diabetes.

Hypoglycemia

Hypoglycemia is also known as "low blood sugar." Reactive hypoglycemia is almost always caused by eating too much carbohydrate. Eating too much carbohydrate elevates blood sugar levels (hyperglycemia) and, when blood sugar rises too much or too fast, insulin is released to lower it. The problem occurs when insulin drives blood sugar too low. The brain is deprived of its sole source of fuel, and hypoglycemic symptoms such as fatigue, rapid heartbeat, sweating, hunger, trembling, headache, mental dullness, and confusion set in. Unlike a high-carbohydrate diet, *40-30-30 Fat-Burning Nutrition* can help keep blood sugar balanced, thus helping to avoid hypoglycemia.

High Blood Pressure

Elevated insulin levels trigger "bad" eicosanoid production which can cause blood vessels to constrict (vasoconstriction) and increase blood pressure. *40-30-30 Fat-Burning Nutrition* helps keep blood sugar balanced, controlling insulin's negative response. This can reduce your risk of high blood pressure.

High Cholesterol

Elevated insulin levels activate the enzyme HMG CoA reductase which can cause the liver to make more cholesterol. No matter how low your diet is in cholesterol, elevated insulin levels can keep your cholesterol levels high. On the other hand, glucagon inhibits the activation of HMG CoA, thereby reducing the amount of cholesterol the liver makes.

40-30-30 Fat-Burning Nutrition can help keep blood sugar stable, elevate glucagon to control cholesterol synthesis, and provide the nutritional support that you need to help reduce high cholesterol levels.

Cancer and Your Immune System

Your body's main defense against cancer is your immune system. Elevated insulin levels suppress your immune system by stimulating the production of the "bad" eicosanoid hormone, PGE2. This hormone inhibits the activation of natural killer cells and decreases oxygen transfer. *40-30-30 Fat-Burning Nutrition* can help in your fight against cancer by elevating glucagon and helping to control insulin, which will minimize the production of PGE2. Also, *40-30-30 Fat-Burning Nutrition* food recommendations are nutrient dense and high in the antioxidant vitamins, which are your body's powerful cell protectors. *40-30-30 Fat-Burning Nutrition* should be the first line of defense for any cancer patient and a key preventative measure for everyone else.

Premenstrual Syndrome (PMS)

Many of the symptoms associated with PMS are directly related to elevated blood glucose levels. By using *40-30-30 Fat-Burning Nutrition*, you can help to control high blood sugar, thus eliminating many of the monthly nightmares associated with PMS. Remember that *40-30-30 Fat-Burning Nutrition* can help control powerful hormonal responses in the body that ultimately control an even wider range of hormonal responses—particularly female hormonal imbalances.

Depression and Mood Swings

A high-carbohydrate diet can lead to protein and amino acid deficiencies that can lead to decreased neurotransmitter production as well as increased insulin production. This ultimately creates a cascade of hormonal responses responsible for the uptake and release of the neurotransmitters. If the brain has low levels of neurotransmitters *or* poor uptake and release of neurotransmitters, depression quickly sets in. *40-30-30 Fat-Burning Nutrition* can provide adequate amounts of quality protein that supply the amino acid precursors for your neurotransmitters. *40-30-30 Fat-Burning Nutrition* can also improve the function of your biological switches providing nutritional support to help control depression and mood swings.

Sleep Disorders

When you eat a high-carbohydrate snack prior to bedtime, you can cause blood sugar and insulin levels to surge. Elevated insulin during sleep not only blocks HGH (human growth hormone) release, inhibiting proper repair and recovery of your body, but you'll find that you may wake up groggy and need even more sleep. You may also experience low blood sugar, which can cause disrupted sleep patterns and waking after only a few hours of sleep.

But eating a *40-30-30 Fat-Burning Nutrition* snack before bed can stabilize blood sugar and trigger the hormonal response to release maximum levels of HGH for body repair, as well as improve sleep patterns to ensure that you wake up bright and alert.

Difficulty Gaining Weight

For those individuals who can't seem to gain weight no matter *what* they eat, *40-30-30 Fat-Burning Nutrition* can be *very* beneficial. To gain weight (muscle, not fat) you need to maximize your body's production of HGH, the body's most powerful muscle building hormone. You also need to provide adequate amounts of protein and amino acids to build and repair muscle tissue. Elevated insulin can inhibit the release of HGH from the pituitary gland. *40-30-30 Fat-Burning Nutrition* is designed to help keep blood sugar levels stable, thereby maximizing the release of glucagon and HGH while providing adequate amounts of protein and amino acids for muscle tissue growth and repair. To gain muscle weight, simply start by adding one additional 40-30-30 meal to your meal planner each day.

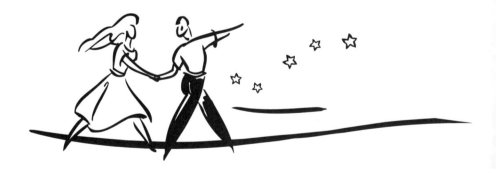

ADJUSTING 40-30-30 FAT-BURNING NUTRITION

The good news about vegetarian diets is that they can be very healthy (high in vitamins, minerals, and fiber) and, with minor adjustments, you can apply the *40-30-30 Fat-Burning Nutrition* principles to create a more balanced vegetarian diet while you maximize your body's ability to burn stored body fat for energy. The bad news about vegetarian diets is that they are typically too high in carbohydrates and low in quality proteins, spiking blood sugar up and making fat burning more difficult.

At the BioSyn Human Performance Center, we worked with hundreds of vegetarians. In most cases, they had a high fat-to-muscle ratio. Even those who were thin still had a high percentage of body fat and were losing lean muscle mass. The reason was pretty obvious. Most vegetarian diets are high in carbohydrate (pasta, potatoes, beans, rice, and bread) and low in quality protein. Those clients were stimulating too much insulin and not burning body fat. To make matters worse, since they were not eating adequate amounts of quality protein, many were losing muscle, slowing their metabolism and fat burning down to a trickle.

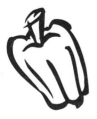

With a few changes you can modify any diet, including vegetarian diets, to adhere to the *40-30-30 Fat-Burning Nutrition* guidelines and maximize the burning of stored body fat.

THE THREE BASIC TYPES OF VEGETARIAN DIETS

Vegans

These are the strict or true vegetarians who eat no animal products, only plant source foods.

40-30-30 Fat-Burning Nutrition Adjustments. A vegan diet is the hardest of all vegetarian diets to balance since it is so high in carbohydrates and low in quality proteins. To balance a vegan diet, simply decrease the amount of starches at each meal (grains, breads, pasta, potatoes, etc.), and increase low-glycemic fruits and vegetables. Add to each meal a large serving of an appropriate low-fat, low-carbohydrate, high-quality vegetarian protein, such as low-fat tofu, tempeh, soy meat substitutes or soy protein powder. Your choices are somewhat limited, but take the time to shop your local health food store to find some of the many new high-protein items made from soy.

Lacto Vegetarians

Lacto vegetarians do not eat animal meat or eggs, but will eat dairy products and food from plant sources.

40-30-30 Fat-Burning Nutrition Adjustments. Lacto vegetarian diets are also very high in carbohydrates. To balance a lacto vegetarian diet, decrease the amount of starches and increase the amount of low-glycemic fruits and vegetables. Add to each meal a large serving of an appropriate low-fat, low-carbohydrate, high-quality protein like cottage cheese, low-fat hard or soft cheese, low-fat tofu and tempeh, soy meat substitutes, or soy and whey protein powders.

> *Most vegetarian diets are high in carbohydrates and low in quality protein. With a few changes you can modify any diet...and maximize the burning of stored body fat.*

Ovolacto Vegetarians

Ovolacto vegetarians do not eat animal meat, but will eat eggs, dairy products, and foods from plant sources.

40-30-30 Fat-Burning Nutrition Adjustments. Ovolacto vegetarian diets are the easiest of all vegetarian diets to balance. Decrease the amount of starches and increase the amount of low-glycemic fruits and vegetables. Add to each meal a large serving of an appropriate low-fat, low-carbohydrate, high-quality protein like cottage cheese, low-fat hard or soft cheese, eggs, egg whites, tofu or tempeh, soy meat substitutes and soy, egg and milk, or whey protein powders.

For more information, see Chapter 8, "Putting It All Together" for individual vegetarian meal guidelines.

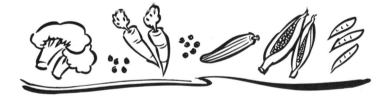

Putting It All Together

(Simply Choose the Appropriate Meal Planner)

BODY WEIGHT
The bigger you are
the more food you need

+

ACTIVITY LEVELS
The more active or stressed you are
the more nutrition you need

=

YOUR PERSONAL REQUIREMENTS
Choose meal planner
A, B, C or D

CHOOSING YOUR MEAL PLANNER

Your body size and activity level determines the overall amount of food and calories you need daily to maximize the burning of stored body fat for energy. One program would never work for everyone. There are four different sizes of the *40-30-30 Fat-Burning Nutrition* meal planners (A, B, C, and D). This allows you to choose the right amount of food to address your approximate needs, but all contain the same *40-30-30 Fat-Burning Nutrition* ratio. Each meal and recipe has been specifically designed to contain 40 percent of the calories from carbohydrate, 30 percent from protein, and 30 percent or less from fat.

Use the conversion chart on the next page to choose the correct meal planner for your size. Find your activity level, the hours you work out per week, and your weight to determine the meal planner that is right for you.

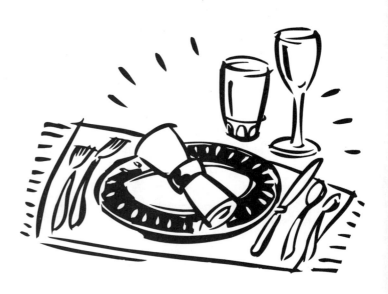

Meal Planner Conversion Chart

WOMEN		
ACTIVITY LEVEL (Hours Per Week of Exercise)	LOW - MEDIUM 0 - 4 HOURS Use Meal Planner	MEDIUM - HIGH 5 -10 HOURS Use Meal Planner
Weight Under 140 lbs	A	B
141 - 180 lbs	B	C
181 - 200+ lbs	C	D

MEN		
ACTIVITY LEVEL (Hours Per Week of Exercise)	LOW - MEDIUM 0 - 4 HOURS Use Meal Planner	MEDIUM - HIGH 5 -10 HOURS Use Meal Planner
Weight Under 140 lbs	B	C
141 - 180 lbs	C	D
181 - 250+ lbs	C	D

If you are a competitive athlete or are very active, choose the next higher meal planner / or add one additional meal per day.

We have provided you with delicious and easy-to-prepare meal planners that show you exactly how much carbohydrate, protein, and fat you need at each meal.

Your Meal Planner is: _____

Build Your Own 40-30-30 Fat-Burning Nutrition Meal

We have provided you with delicious and easy-to-prepare meal planners on the following pages that show you exactly how much carbohydrate, protein, and fat you need at each meal and snack per day.

Your breakfast, lunch, snack, and dinner requirements are listed on the following page. Typical American eating habits usually dictate a smaller breakfast and lunch, and a larger dinner. If you prefer to have a larger meal at lunchtime and a smaller dinner, by all means do.

Our goal is to teach you how to eat the correct *40-30-30 Fat-Burning Nutrition* ratio at every meal and snack. We have provided meal examples for you to use to get a better idea of what a *40-30-30 Fat-Burning Nutrition* meal should look like. With a little practice, you will see how simple it is to prepare an infinite amount of meal and snack choices. Use *Your 40-30-30 Fat-Burning Nutrition Requirements* listed on the next page to determine how much carbohydrate, protein, and fat you need at each meal. Then, using The Glycemic Index in Chapter 4,

Using the Glycemic Index in Chapter 4, the Food Value Guide in Chapter 11, and the Restaurants, Prepared Foods, and Fast Food Guide in Chapter 12, you can begin to prepare an unlimited variety of meals, snacks, and recipes on your own.

The Food Value Guide in Chapter 11, and the Restaurants, Prepared Foods, and Fast Food Guide in Chapter 12, you can begin to prepare an unlimited variety of meals, snacks, and recipes on your own.

NOTE: Fat-Burning Nutrition Proportion Chart is listed in the appendix.

Your 40-30-30 Fat-Burning Nutrition Requirements

| | AMOUNT FOR MEAL PLANNERS | | | |
	A	B	C	D
BREAKFAST				
Carbohydrate	20 g	20 g	33 g	47 g
Protein	15 g	15 g	25 g	35 g
Fat	6 g	6 g	11 g	13 g
LUNCH				
Carbohydrate	27 g	40 g	40 g	53 g
Protein	20 g	30 g	30 g	40 g
Fat	9 g	14 g	14 g	18 g
SNACK				
Carbohydrate	20 g	20 g	20 g	20 g
Protein	15 g	15 g	15 g	15 g
Fat	6 g	6 g	6 g	6 g
DINNER				
Carbohydrate	40 g	47 g	53 g	53 g
Protein	30 g	35 g	40 g	40 g
Fat	14 g	15 g	18 g	18 g

* g=grams

** We recommend a 40-30-30 meal replacement bar for snacks or as a complete breakfast or lunch when you don't have time to make a balanced 40-30-30 meal. Most bars on the market are very high in carbohydrate, so make sure you read the label to see that they contain only 1/3 more carbohydrate than protein <u>and</u> some fat. A 40-30-30 ratio for a nutrition bar should contain approximately 20 grams of carbohydrate,15 grams of protein, and 6 grams of fat.

Sample Starter Meal Planners

We have provided you with Sample Starter Meal Planners containing simple-to-prepare meals that follow the 40-30-30 ratio. Included are the *FBN Regular Meals, FBN Fat-Flush Meals,* and *FBN Vegetarian Meals.* The daily order of the menu is not important, but the amount of carbohydrate, protein, and fat is. If you do not like a sample meal on a particular day, find one that you <u>do</u> like and use it. Don't skip meals in an attempt to speed up the fat-burning process. Missed meals or snacks can actually slow your metabolism and the fat-loss process. It is important to choose the correct meal planner for your size to feed your body properly.

R
E
G
U
L
A
R

MEALS

FBN REGULAR MEALS

FBN Regular Meals are well-balanced meals and snacks with the 40-30-30 ratio. They are designed with a variety of high- and low-glycemic carbohydrates, quality protein, and fat. We are sure you will find them to be delicious and easy to prepare.

Snacks have also been provided as part of your daily dietary requirements. Since lunch is not intended to control appetite longer than 4-5 hours, a small snack is required mid-afternoon. It will help to provide stable energy levels all afternoon and help to eliminate overeating at dinner. We also recommend the use of a 40-30-30 Nutrition bar for convenient mid-afternoon snacks. 40-30-30 Nutrition bars can also be used for breakfast or lunch when you don't have time for a well balanced meal. However, you should limit the Nutrition bars to no more than two per day.

40-30-30 Nutrition bars can also be used for breakfast or lunch when you don't have time for a well balanced meal. However, you should limit the Nutrition bars to no more than two per day.

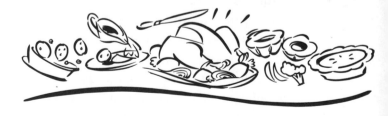

FBN Regular Meals—Example Day 1

AMOUNTS FOR MEAL PLANNERS

BREAKFAST	A	B	C	D
Fruit Protein Shake				
Protein Powder (1 scoop = 16 g)	1	1	2	2 1/4
Banana, medium, frozen	1/2	1/2	2/3	1
Strawberries, frozen	1/2 c.	1/2 c.	1 c.	1 c.
Water	3/4 c.	3/4 c.	1 c.	11/4 c.
Almonds, raw	2 t.	2 t.	1 T.	2 T.
Honey	0	0	1 tsp.	2 tsp.

Directions: *Combine all ingredients in a high-speed blender and blend till smooth.*

LUNCH	A	B	C	D
Turkey Sandwich				
Wheat Bread, whole grain	1 slice	2 slices	2 slices	2 slices
Turkey Breast, sliced	1 1/2 oz.	3 oz.	3 oz.	4 oz.
Lettuce, leaf	1	1	1	1
Tomato Slice	1	1	1	2
Mayonnaise, reduced-fat	1 T.	1 1/2 T.	1 1/2 T.	2 T.
Fruit	1 plum	1 plum	1 plum	1 apple

Directions: *Prepare turkey sandwich and serve with fruit and beverage.*

SNACK	A	B	C	D
Turkey Bagel				
Mini bagel	1	1	1	1
Turkey breast, sliced	1 1/2 oz	1 1/2 oz.	1 1/2 oz.	1 1/2 oz.
Cream cheese, whipped, low-fat	1/2 oz.	1/2 oz.	1/2 oz.	1/2 oz.

Directions: *Spread cream cheese on bagel halves and top with turkey.*

Or a 40-30-30 Nutrition Bar	**1 bar**	**1 bar**	**1 bar**	**1 bar**

DINNER	A	B	C	D
Easy Pizza at Home				
Tortilla, flour 8-9"	1	1 1/2	2	2
Pizza Sauce	3 T.	4 T.	6 T.	6 T.
Chicken Strips, precooked	2.5 oz.	3.5 oz.	4 oz.	4 oz.
Mixed Vegetables (onions, red or green peppers, mushrooms), sliced	1 c.	1 1/4 c.	1 1/2 c.	1 1/2 c.
Mozzarella Cheese, low-fat	1 oz.	1 oz.	1 1/2 oz.	1 1/2 oz
Green Salad	2 c.	2 c.	3 c.	3 c.
Italian Salad Dressing*	1 T.	1 T.	2 T.	2 T.

Directions: *Top tortilla with pizza sauce, chicken, mixed vegetables and cheese. Bake in 400° oven till cheese is melted and lightly browned. Serve with a green salad and Italian dressing.*

* Italian Dressing recipe: Combine 1 T. olive oil, 1 T. red wine vinegar and 1 t. lemon juice in a small jar. Add salt, pepper, fresh garlic or garlic powder to taste. Shake well.

■ Beverages: Always consume an 8 oz. appropriate beverage with each meal (see Chapter 9).

■ Nutrition bar: A 40-30-30 Nutrition Bar may be substituted for breakfast, lunch, or snack when desired.

R
E
G
U
L
A
R

MEALS

FBN Regular Meals—Example Day 2

AMOUNT FOR MEAL PLANNERS

BREAKFAST	A	B	C	D
Hot Cereal and Cottage Cheese				
Oatmeal, slow cooked in water	1/2 c.	1/2 c.	1 c.	1 1/4 c.
Milk, non-fat	1/4 c.	1/4 c.	1/2 c.	1/2 c.
Almonds, raw	1 t.	1 t.	2 t.	1 T.
Brown Sugar or Honey	1 t.	1 t.	1 t.	1 t.
Cottage Cheese, 2% low-fat	1/3 c.	1/3 c.	1/2 c.	3/4 c.

Directions: *Cook oatmeal and top with milk, almonds, and sugar. Stir in cottage cheese or have it on the side.*

LUNCH	A	B	C	D
Tuna Pita Pocket with Fruit				
Albacore Tuna,				
water packed, drained	3 oz.	4 oz.	4 oz.	5 oz.
Sweet Pickle Relish	1 t.	1 t.	1 t.	1 T.
Celery Stalk, chopped	1/2	1/2	1/2	1/2
Onion, chopped	1 T.	1 T.	1 T.	1 T.
Mayonnaise, reduced-fat	1 T.	2 T.	2 T.	3 T.
Pita Pocket, wheat or white	1/2	3/4	3/4	1
Grapes, green or red, seedless	15	20	20	20

Directions: *Combine tuna with pickles, celery, onion, and mayonnaise. Place in pita pocket bread and serve with grapes.*

SNACK	A	B	C	D
String Cheese and Apple				
String Cheese, low-fat, 1 oz.	1	1	1	1
Apple, small	1	1	1	1

Directions: *Have string cheese with a small apple.*

Or a 40-30-30 Nutrition Bar	**1 bar**	**1 bar**	**1 bar**	**1 bar**

DINNER	A	B	C	D
Steak and Potatoes				
Top Sirloin or Filet Mignon, lean	3 oz.	4 oz.	5 oz.	5 oz.
New Potatoes, red, 1 1/2" diameter	2	3	3	3
Broccoli, steamed	1 c.	1 1/2 c.	2 c.	2 c.
Green Salad	2 c.	3 c.	3 c.	3 c.
Salad Dressing, low-fat or fat-free	2 t.	2 t.	1 T.	1 T.

Directions: *Grill steak. Serve with steamed little red potatoes and broccoli and a large green salad. Use a fat-free or reduced-fat salad dressing since steak contains fat.*

- Beverages: Always consume an 8 oz. appropriate beverage with each meal (see Chapter 9).
- Nutrition bar: A 40-30-30 Nutrition Bar may be substituted for breakfast, lunch, or snack when desired.

FBN Regular Meals—Example Day 3

AMOUNT FOR MEAL PLANNERS

BREAKFAST	A	B	C	D
Egg and Cheese Burrito				
Tortilla, fat-free 7-8", flour	1	1	2	2
Eggs, whole	1	1	2	2
Egg whites	1	1	3	5
Cheddar cheese, low-fat	1/2 oz.	1/2 oz.	1 oz.	1 1/2 oz
Salsa	1 T.	1 T.	2 T.	3 T.

Directions: *Scramble eggs, roll in tortilla with cheese and salsa.*

LUNCH	A	B	C	D
Fruit Protein Shake				
Whey Protein Powder				
(1 scoop = 16 g)	1	11/2	11/2	2
Banana, medium, frozen	1/2	1/2	1/2	1
Peaches, frozen	1/2 c.	1 c.	1 c.	1 c.
Water	3/4 c.	1 c.	1 c.	1 1/4 c.
Walnuts, raw	1 T.	1 1/2 T.	1 1/2 T.	2 T.

Directions: *Combine all ingredients in a high-speed blender and blend till smooth.*

SNACK	A	B	C	D
Tortilla Turkey Roll Up				
Tortilla, 7", flour	1	1	1	1
Turkey Breast, sliced	2.5 oz.	2.5 oz.	2.5 oz.	2.5 oz.

Directions: *Place turkey in tortilla, roll and eat.*

Or a 40-30-30 Nutrition Bar	**1 bar**	**1 bar**	**1 bar**	**1 bar**

DINNER	A	B	C	D
Grilled Teriyaki Chicken Dinner				
Chicken Breast,				
in teriyaki marinade*	3 oz.	4 oz.	4.5 oz.	4.5 oz.
Brown Rice, cooked	1/2 c.	1/2 c.	2/3 c.	2/3 c.
Green Beans	1 c.	1 c.	1 1/2 c.	1 1/2 c.
Peaches, fresh or water packed	1/2 c.	2/3 c.	2/3 c.	2/3 c.

Directions: *Marinate skinless chicken breast in teriyaki sauce. Broil or grill chicken and baste during cooking. Serve with brown rice (flavor to taste with soy sauce), green beans, and peaches for dessert.*

* Teriyaki Marinade recipe: Combine 2 T. vegetable oil, 2 T. soy sauce, 2 t. brown sugar, 1/2 t. garlic powder and 1/2 T. sherry. Add chicken and marinate for several hours. (You may use 2 1/2 T. of bottled Teriyaki marinade).

■ Beverages: Always consume an 8 oz. appropriate beverage with each meal (see Chapter 9).

■ Nutrition bar: A 40-30-30 Nutrition Bar may be substituted for breakfast, lunch, or snack when desired.

R
E
G
U
L
A
R

MEALS

FBN Regular Meals—Example Day 4

AMOUNT FOR MEAL PLANNERS

BREAKFAST **Bagel Breakfast Sandwich**	A	B	C	D
Bagel	1/2	1/2	1 large	2 med.
Cream Cheese, low-fat, whipped	2 t.	2 t.	1 T.	2 T.
Turkey Breast, sliced	2 oz.	2 oz.	4 oz.	5 oz.

Directions: *Place cream cheese and turkey on bagel.*

LUNCH **Roast Beef Sandwich**	A	B	C	D
Bread, rye	1	2	2	2
Roast Beef, lean	3 oz.	5 oz.	5 oz.	6 oz.
Dijonnaise	2 t.	1 T.	1 T.	1 1/2 T.
Lettuce, leaf	1	2	2	2
Tomato Slice	1	1	1	2
Pretzel Sticks, (22 sticks per ounce)	1/2 oz.	1/2 oz.	1/2 oz.	1 oz.

Directions: *Spread Dijonnaise on rye bread and top with roast beef, lettuce, and tomato. Serve sandwich with pretzel sticks.*

SNACK **Small Peanut Butter Protein Shake**	A	B	C	D
Whey Protein Powder (1 scoop = 16 g)	1	1	1	1
Banana, frozen	1/2	1/2	1/2	1/2
Peanut Butter, all natural	1 T.	1 T.	1 T.	1 T.
Water	1/2 c.	1/2 c.	1/2 c.	1/2 c.

Directions: *Combine all ingredients in a high-speed blender and blend till smooth.*

Or a 40-30-30 Nutrition Bar	1 bar	1 bar	1 bar	1 bar

DINNER **Tuna Pasta Caesar Salad**	A	B	C	D
Romaine Lettuce	1/2 head	1/2 head	1/2 head	1/2 head
Tortellini, cooked	1 oz.	1 1/2 oz.	2 oz.	2 oz.
Albacore Tuna, water packed, drain	2 oz.	2 1/2 oz.	3 oz.	3 oz.
Croutons	1/2 oz.	1/2 oz.	1/2 oz.	1/2 oz.
Parmesan Cheese, grated	1 T.	1 1/2 T.	2 T.	2 T.
Caesar Salad Dressing*				

Directions: *Clean, dry, and tear romaine lettuce. Add tuna and cooked and cooled tortellini. Toss with Caesar salad dressing and top with croutons and grated parmesan cheese.*

* Caesar Salad Dressing recipe: One serving. Recipe can be doubled or tripled. 1 T. olive oil (extra virgin), 1 T. red wine vinegar, 1/2 T. fresh lemon juice, 1 small clove garlic, pressed, 1/2 t. Worcestershire sauce, 1/2 t. anchovy paste, 1/4 t. dry mustard, 1/4 t. fresh ground pepper, 1/8 t. salt (optional). Place all ingredients in a small glass jar and shake well.

■ Beverages: Always consume an 8 oz. appropriate beverage with each meal (see Chapter 9).

■ Nutrition bar: A 40-30-30 Nutrition Bar may be substituted for breakfast, lunch, or snack when desired.

FBN Regular Meals—Example Day 5

AMOUNT FOR MEAL PLANNERS

BREAKFAST	A	B	C	D
Fresh Fruit and Cottage Cheese				
Cottage Cheese, 2% low-fat	1/2 c.	1/2 c.	1 c.	11/4 c.
Apple	1 small	1 small	1 large	2 med.
Walnuts, raw	2 t.	2 t.	1 T.	1 1/2 T.

Directions: *Serve cottage cheese with sliced apple and walnuts.*

LUNCH	A	B	C	D
Bagel Sandwich				
Bagel	1/2	1	1	1
Turkey or Chicken Breast, sliced	2 1/2 oz.	4 oz.	4 oz.	5 oz.
Lettuce, leaf	1	1	1	2
Tomato slice	1	1	1	2
Mayonnaise, reduced-calorie	1 T.	2 T.	2 T.	2 T.
Tangerine				

Directions: *Spread mayonnaise on bagel. Top with sliced turkey or chicken, lettuce, and tomato. Serve with fruit.*

SNACK	A	B	C	D
Cottage Cheese and Pineapple				
Cottage Cheese				
with pineapple, 4 oz.	1	1	1	1

Directions: *Buy prepared low-fat cottage cheese with pineapple added.*

Or a 40-30-30 Nutrition Bar	**1 bar**	**1 bar**	**1 bar**	**1 bar**

DINNER	A	B	C	D
Grilled Fish Dinner				
Salmon, broiled or grilled	3 1/2 oz.	4 oz.	4 1/2 oz.	4 1/2 oz.
Brown Rice, cooked	1/2 c.	1/2 c.	2/3 c.	2/3 c.
Asparagus Spears	8	8	10	10
Dinner Salad	1 c.	2 c.	2 c.	2 c.
Salad Dressing, full-fat, your choice	2 t.	1 T.	1 1/2 T.	1 1/2 T.
Pears, fresh or water packed	1/2 c.	1/2 c.	1/2 c.	1/2 c.

Directions: *Grill salmon steak seasoned with fresh lemon and dill. Serve with brown rice, steamed fresh asparagus spears, dinner salad with salad dressing and pears for dessert.*

■ Beverages: Always consume an 8 oz. appropriate beverage with each meal (see Chapter 9).

■ Nutrition bar: A 40-30-30 Nutrition Bar may be substituted for breakfast, lunch, or snack when desired.

FBN Regular Meals—Example Day 6

REGULAR

MEALS

	AMOUNT FOR MEAL PLANNERS			
BREAKFAST	A	B	C	D
Scrambled Eggs and Toast				
Eggs, whole	1	1	2	2
Egg Whites	1	1	3	5
Cheddar Cheese, low-fat	1/2 oz.	1/2 oz.	1 oz.	1 oz.
Whole Wheat Toast	1 slice	1 slice	2 slices	2 slices
Orange	1/2	1/2	1/2	1

Directions: *Scramble eggs, top with cheese. Serve with toast and orange slices.*

LUNCH	A	B	C	D
Fruit Salad with Cottage Cheese				
Lettuce leaves	2	2	2	3
Cottage Cheese, 2% low-fat	2/3 c.	1 c.	1 c.	1 1/3 c.
Pineapple	1/4 c.	1/2 c.	1/2 c.	1/2 c.
Apple	1 small	1 medium	1 medium	1 large
Walnuts or Almonds, raw	2 t.	1 T.	1 T.	1 1/2 T.

Directions: *Place cottage cheese, pineapple and sliced apple on a bed of lettuce. Sprinkle with nuts.*

SNACK	A	B	C	D
Tuna on Rye Crackers				
Albacore Tuna, water packed, drain	2	2	2	2
Mayonnaise, safflower	1 t.	1 t.	1 t.	1 t.
Rye Crackers, (Rykrisp)	2	2	2	2

Directions: *Mix tuna with mayonnaise and serve on crackers.*

Or a 40-30-30 Nutrition Bar	**1 bar**	**1 bar**	**1 bar**	**1 bar**

DINNER	A	B	C	D
Hearty Chili				
Hearty Chili* (see recipe)	1 1/2 c.	2 c.	2 1/2 c.	2 1/2 c.
Small Oyster Crackers	10	15	20	20
Green Salad	1 c.	1 c.	2 c.	2 c.
Salad Dressing, full-fat	2 t.	1 T.	1 1/2 T.	1 1/2 T.

Directions: *Enjoy a bowl of chili with crackers, dinner salad, and a full-fat salad dressing of your choice.*

* Hearty Chili recipe: Brown 1 pound of ground turkey breast or extra-lean ground beef. Add 1/2 c. chopped celery, 1 c. chopped green pepper, 1 c. chopped onion, 1/2 c. fresh parsley, and 1 c. chopped mushrooms. Stir in 1 package chili seasonings. Add 14.5 oz. canned tomatoes with juice, 15 oz. canned tomato sauce, 8 oz. can tomato puree, and a 15 oz. can of black beans. Mix well and simmer for at least one hour. If you like your chili spicy, add 1/2 - 1 t. crushed red pepper flakes.

■ Beverages: Always consume an 8 oz. appropriate beverage with each meal (see Chapter 9).

■ Nutrition bar: A 40-30-30 Nutrition Bar may be substituted for breakfast, lunch, or snack when desired.

FBN Regular Meals—Example Day 7

AMOUNT FOR MEAL PLANNERS

BREAKFAST	A	B	C	D
Open Face Ham Sandwich				
English Muffin Halves, toasted	1	1	2	3
Breakfast Ham, lean	2 oz.	2 oz.	2 1/2 oz.	4 oz.
Mozzarella Cheese, part skim	1/2 oz.	1/2 oz.	1 oz.	1 oz.
Tangerine	1	1	1	1

Directions: *Place ham and cheese on a toasted muffin half and broil till hot. Serve with a tangerine.*

LUNCH	A	B	C	D
Grilled Chicken Sandwich				
Hamburger Bun	1*	1	1	1
Chicken Breast	2.5 oz.	3.5 oz.	3.5 oz.	4.5 oz.
Lettuce, leaf	1	1	1	2
Mayonnaise, reduced-fat	2 t.	1 T.	1 T.	1 T.
Side Salad	1 small	1 large	1 large	1 large
Salad Dressing, low-fat	2 t.	1 T.	1 T.	2 T.

Directions: *Serve grilled chicken breast on hamburger bun with lettuce and mayonnaise. Serve with a side salad and low-fat salad dressing.*

SNACK	A	B	C	D
Shrimp Cocktail				
Shrimp, large, cooked	12	12	12	12
Cocktail Sauce	1/4 c.	1/4 c.	1/4 c.	1/4 c.

Directions: *Shell and devein cooked shrimp. Serve with prepared cocktail sauce.*

Or a 40-30-30 Nutrition Bar	1 bar	1 bar	1 bar	1 bar

DINNER	A	B	C	D
Shredded Beef Burritos				
Beef Mixture** (see recipe)	4 oz.	5 oz.	6 oz.	6 oz.
Tortilla, flour, 8" size	1 1/2	2	2 1/2	2 1/2
Lettuce, shredded	1/2 c.	3/4 c.	1 c.	1 c.
Tomato, chopped	2 T.	3 T.	4 T.	4 T.
Salsa	2-3 T.	3-4 T.	4-5 T.	4-5 T.
Sour Cream, low-fat	1 T.	2 T.	2 T.	2 T.

Directions: *Place sour cream and shredded beef on a warm flour tortilla, top with lettuce, tomato, and salsa. Fold burrito style and serve topped with additional shredded lettuce and salsa.*

* Reduced Calorie

** Shredded Beef recipe: Trim and discard all visible fat from 2 pounds of beef and place in 5-6 qt. pan with 1/4 c. water. Cover and cook over medium heat for 30 minutes. Uncover and cook until liquid evaporates and meat is well browned. In a bowl, combine 3 T. red wine vinegar, 1 1/2 c. regular-strength chicken broth, 2 T. chili powder, 1 t. ground cumin. Mix well and pour over meat. Continue cooking over medium heat until meat is very tender and pulls apart easily (about two hours). Let meat cool, then shred with two forks and mix with pan juices.

■ Beverages: Always consume an 8 oz. appropriate beverage with each meal (see Chapter 9).

■ Nutrition bar: A 40-30-30 Nutrition Bar may be substituted for breakfast, lunch, or snack when desired.

R
E
G
U
L
A
R

MEALS

FBN FAT-FLUSH MEALS

FBN Fat-Flush Meals are more strictly structured than the *Regular FBN Meals* for those who want to accelerate fat loss to near genetic maximum rates. This accelerated plan follows the *40-30-30 Fat-Burning Nutrition* ratio and contains only low-glycemic carbohydrate sources from fruits and vegetables (no starches or refined sugars), with quality protein and fat.

You can use *FBN Fat-Flush Meals* daily for several weeks at a time. Our *Two-Week Fat-Flush* program promotes using these meals for two weeks, back to back. By completely eliminating high-glycemic carbohydrate from your diet, the fastest results can be expected. You will find that after that time, you will begin to miss the higher-glycemic carbohydrate and want to alternate these meals with the *Regular FBN Meals* containing some starches.

> By completely eliminating high-glycemic carbohydrate the fastest results can be expected. You'll never feel sluggish after a FBN Fat-Flush Meal.

Use the *FBN Fat-Flush Meals* any time you want to really kick up your ability to burn fat another notch. They contain plenty of high-fiber foods, are easy to prepare, and taste great. You'll never feel sluggish after a *FBN Fat-Flush Meal*.

Mid-afternoon snacks have also been included since lunch is not intended to control appetite longer than 4-5 hours. You may use a 40-30-30 Nutrition Bar on the *FBN Fat-Flush* plan in place of the snack. Even though a 40-30-30 Nutrition Bar contains several sources of carbohydrate (sugars), they also contain the precise amount of protein and fat to control blood sugar levels and produce an overall low-glycemic response.

FAT FLUSH MEALS

FBN Fat-Flush Meals—Example Day 1

AMOUNT FOR MEAL PLANNERS

BREAKFAST	A	B	C	D
Scrambled Eggs and Fruit				
Eggs, whole	1	1	2	3
Egg Whites	2	2	3	4
Tomato, 2.6" diameter	1	1	1	2
Orange	1 medium	1 medium	1 large	1 large

Directions: *Crack eggs and discard some of the yolks. Scramble and serve with sliced tomato and an orange.*

LUNCH	A	B	C	D
Tuna Salad				
Albacore Tuna, in water, drained	3 oz.	4 oz.	4 oz.	6 oz.
Sweet Pickle Relish	1 T.	1 T.	1 T.	2 T.
Celery, diced	3 T.	3 T.	3 T.	5 T.
Grapes, seedless	10	15	15	20
Mayonnaise, safflower	2 t.	1 T.	1 T.	1 1/2 T.
Lettuce Leaves	2	2	2	4
Apple	1/2	1	1	1 large

Directions: *Prepare tuna salad by combining tuna, pickle relish, celery, grapes, and mayonnaise. Serve on lettuce leaves and crisp apple slices.*

SNACK	A	B	C	D
Cottage Cheese with Pineapple				
Cottage Cheese with Pineapple, 4 oz.	1	1	1	1

Directions: *Buy prepared low-fat cottage cheese with pineapple added.*

Or a 40-30-30 Nutrition Bar	**1 bar**	**1 bar**	**1 bar**	**1 bar**

DINNER	A	B	C	D
Barbecued Chicken				
Chicken Breast	3.5 oz.	4.5 oz.	5 oz.	5 oz.
Barbecue Sauce	1 T.	2 T.	2 T.	2 T.
Cabbage, grated	1 c.	1 c.	1 1/2 c.	1 1/2 c.
Coleslaw Dressing, bottled	1 T.	1 T.	1 1/2 T.	1 1/2 T.
Pineapple Rings (grilled)	2	2	3	3
Green Beans	1 c.	1 c.	1 c.	1 c.

Directions: *Grill chicken breast and baste with barbecue sauce. Combine cabbage and coleslaw dressing. Serve with green beans and grilled pineapple rings.*

■ Beverages: Always consume an 8 oz. appropriate beverage with each meal (see Chapter 9).

■ Nutrition bar: A 40-30-30 Nutrition Bar may be substituted for breakfast, lunch, or snack when desired.

**F
A
T

F
L
U
S
H**

MEALS

FBN Fat-Flush Meals—Example Day 2

AMOUNT FOR MEAL PLANNERS

BREAKFAST	A	B	C	D
Cottage Cheese and Fruit				
Cottage Cheese, 2% low-fat	1/2 c.	1/2 c.	3/4 c.	1 c.
Peaches, fresh or water packed	1 c.	1 c.	2 c.	2 1/2 c.
Almonds, raw	1/2 T.	1/2 T.	1 T.	1 1/2 T.

Directions: *Have cottage cheese with peaches and sprinkle with almonds.*

LUNCH	A	B	C	D
Chicken Caesar Salad				
Romaine Lettuce, cleaned, dried, and torn	2 c.	3 c.	3 c.	4 c.
Chicken, pre-cooked and cooled	2.5 oz.	3.5 oz.	3.5 oz.	4.5 oz.
Caesar Dressing, bottled or see recipe*	2 t.	1 T.	1 T.	1 1/2 T.
Parmesan Cheese, grated	1 t.	1 t.	1 t.	1 t.
Sliced Apple	1 medium	1 large	1 large	1 large

Directions: *Combine romaine lettuce with chicken and Caesar salad dressing. Sprinkle with Parmesan cheese and serve with a fresh sliced apple.*

*Caesar Salad dressing recipe: 1 T. olive oil, 1 T. red wine vinegar, 1/2 T. lemon juice, 1 small clove of garlic, pressed or 1/8 t. garlic powder, 1/2 t. Worcestershire sauce, 1/2 t. anchovy paste, 1/2 t. dry mustard, 1/2 t. fresh ground pepper, 1/8 t. salt (optional). Place all ingredients in a small jar and shake till blended.

SNACK	A	B	C	D
Hard Boiled Eggs and Fruit				
Egg, whole	1	1	1	1
Egg, white	1	1	1	1
Tangerine or Small Orange	1	1	1	1

Directions: *Hard boil eggs. Peel and discard one yolk. Add salt and pepper to taste and eat with an orange.*

Or have a 40-30-30 Nutrition Bar

DINNER	A	B	C	D
Grilled Salmon and Vegetables				
Salmon Steak, grilled	3 1/2 oz.	4 oz.	4 1/2 oz.	4 1/2 oz.
Onions, sweet, large size, thick slices	2	3	3	4
Green Pepper	1/2	1/2	1/2	1
Zucchini	1	1	1	1
Green Salad	1 c.	2 c.	2 c.	2 c.
Salad Dressing, low-fat, your choice	2 t.	1 T.	1 T.	1 T.
Peaches, fresh or water packed	1/2 c.	1 c.	1 c.	1 c.

Directions: *Grill salmon steak with fresh lemon, garlic, salt, and pepper to taste. Grill vegetables; slice a sweet large onion in 1/2" slices, quarter the green pepper and cut zucchini into strips. Serve with a green salad with salad dressing and peaches for dessert.*

■ Beverages: Always consume an 8 oz. appropriate beverage with each meal (see Chapter 9).

■ Nutrition bar: A 40-30-30 Nutrition Bar may be substituted for breakfast, lunch, or snack when desired.

FBN Fat-Flush Meals—Example Day 3

AMOUNT FOR MEAL PLANNERS

BREAKFAST	A	B	C	D
Protein Shake				
Whey Protein Powder				
(1 scoop = 16 g)	1	1	2	2 1/4
Strawberries, fresh or frozen	3/4 c.	3/4 c.	1 c.	1 1/4 c.
Peaches, fresh or frozen	1/2 c.	1/2 c.	2/3 c.	1 c.
Crystalline Fructose*	1 t.	1 t.	1 t.	1 T.
Water	3/4 c.	3/4 c.	1 c.	1 1/2 c.
Almonds	2 t.	2 t.	1 1/2 T.	2 T.

Directions: *Blend all ingredients in a blender and blend till smooth.*

LUNCH	A	B	C	D
Waldorf Turkey Salad				
Turkey Breast, cooked and cooled	2.5 oz.	4 oz.	4 oz.	5 oz.
Celery, diced	2 T.	2 T.	2 T.	3 T.
Grapes, green or red, seedless	10	10	10	20
Apple, diced	1/2	1	1	1 large
Mayonnaise, safflower	2 t.	1 T.	1 T.	1 1/2 T.

Directions: *Cube turkey breast and add to celery, sliced grapes and diced apple. Add mayonnaise with a dash of lemon juice and toss until coated.*

SNACK	A	B	C	D
Sliced Roast Beef and Fruit				
Sliced Roast Beef, lean	2 oz.	2 oz.	2 oz.	2 oz.
Orange, large	1	1	1	1
Directions: *Have lean roast beef with orange.*				
Or a 40-30-30 Nutrition Bar	**1 bar**	**1 bar**	**1 bar**	**1 bar**

DINNER	A	B	C	D
Tuna Plate				
Albacore Tuna,				
water packed, drained	4 oz.	5 oz.	6 oz.	6 oz.
Asparagus Spears,				
cooked and cooled	8	8	10	10
Cucumber Rounds	1/2 c.	1/2 c.	1/2 c.	1/2 c.
Red Leaf Lettuce	4	4	6	6
Applesauce, unsweetened	1/2 c.	1/2 c.	1/2 c.	1/2 c.
Strawberries	1/2 c.	1 c.	1 c.	1 c.
Salad Dressing, lite French	2 T.	2 T.	3 T.	3 T.

Directions: *Place lettuce leaves on plate and top with tuna, asparagus, cucumbers, applesauce and strawberries. Drizzle lite French salad dressing over the lettuce, tuna, asparagus and cucumbers.*

* Crystalline fructose can be bought in most health food stores and is a low-glycemic sweetener.

■ Beverages: Always consume an 8 oz. appropriate beverage with each meal (see Chapter 9).

■ Nutrition bar: A 40-30-30 Nutrition Bar may be substituted for breakfast, lunch, or snack when desired.

FAT FLUSH MEALS

FBN Fat-Flush Meals—Example Day 4

AMOUNT FOR MEAL PLANNERS

BREAKFAST	A	B	C	D
Denver Scramble with Fruit				
Egg, whole	1	1	1	1
Egg Whites	1	1	2	2
Ham, breakfast, X-lean	1 oz.	1 oz.	1.5 oz.	3 oz.
Mushrooms	1 T.	1 T.	2 T.	2 T.
Onion	1 T.	1 T.	1 T.	1 T.
Green pepper	2 T.	2 T.	2 T.	2 T.
Orange Juice	6 oz.	6 oz.	8 oz.	12 oz.

Directions: *Pour blended eggs in a non-stick pan. Add ham, mushrooms, onion, and green peppers. Scramble, sprinkle with salt, pepper, and paprika to taste and serve with orange juice.*

LUNCH	A	B	C	D
Grilled Chicken Breast				
Chicken Breast	2 oz.	3 oz.	3 oz.	5 oz.
Broccoli, steamed	1 c.	1 1/2 c.	1 1/2 c.	2 c.
Applesauce, unsweetened	1/2 c.	3/4 c.	3/4 c.	1 c.
Green Salad, small	1	1	1	1
Salad Dressing, full-fat, your choice	1 T.	1 1/2 T.	1 1/2 T.	2 T.

Directions: *Serve grilled or steamed chicken breast with steamed broccoli, applesauce, and a green salad and salad dressing.*

SNACK	A	B	C	D
String Cheese and Fruit				
String Cheese, low-fat, 1 oz.	1	1	1	1
Apple, small	1	1	1	1
Directions: *Have string cheese with small apple.*				
Or a 40-30-30 Nutrition Bar	**1 bar**	**1 bar**	**1 bar**	**1 bar**

DINNER	A	B	C	D
Beef Tenderloin Dinner				
Beef Tenderloin, extra lean	4 oz.	5 oz.	6 oz.	6 oz.
Asparagus Spears, steamed	8	8	10	10
Tomatoes, stewed	1 c.	1 c.	1 1/2 c.	1 1/2 c.
Green Salad	2 c.	3 c.	4 c.	4 c.
Salad Dressing, low-fat, your choice	2 t.	2 t.	1 T.	1 T.
Pears, fresh or water packed	1 c.	1 c.	1 c.	1 c.

Directions: *Grill or bake the beef tenderloin in foil, seasoned with garlic, salt, and pepper. Serve with fresh steamed asparagus spears, stewed tomatoes, green salad with low-fat dressing and pears for dessert.*

■ Beverages: Always consume an 8 oz. appropriate beverage with each meal (see Chapter 9).

■ Nutrition bar: A 40-30-30 Nutrition Bar may be substituted for breakfast, lunch, or snack when desired.

FBN Fat-Flush Meals—Example Day 5

AMOUNT FOR MEAL PLANNERS

BREAKFAST	A	B	C	D
Yogurt Cheese				
Yogurt, vanilla, low-fat	1/2 c.	1/2 c.	1 c.	1 1/3 c.
Cottage Cheese, 2% low-fat	1/3 c.	1/3 c.	1/2 c.	3/4 c.
Almonds, raw	1 t.	1 t.	2 t.	1 T.

Directions: *Combine yogurt with cottage cheese and top with almonds.*
Note: If using fat-free yogurt or cottage cheese, increase almonds.

LUNCH	A	B	C	D
Pineapple Chicken Salad				
Chicken, cooked, cooled and diced	2.5 oz.	3.5 oz.	3.5 oz.	4.5 oz.
Pineapple Chunks	3/4 c.	1 c.	1 c.	1 1/4 c.
Grapes, sliced	10	15	15	20
Mayonnaise, safflower	2 t.	1 T.	1 T.	1 1/2 T.
Lettuce, shredded	2 c.	3 c.	3 c.	3 c.

Directions: *Blend chicken, pineapple and grapes with mayonnaise. Serve on a bed of shredded lettuce.*

SNACK	A	B	C	D
Small Fruit Protein Shake				
Whey Protein Powder,				
(1 scoop = 16 g)	1	1	1	1
Peaches, frozen	1 c.	1 c.	1 c.	1 c.
Fructose, crystalline	1 t.	1 t.	1 t.	1 t.
Water	1/2 c.	1/2 c.	1/2 c.	1/2 c.
Almonds	2 t.	2 t.	2 t.	2 t.

Directions: *Combine all ingredients in a blender and blend till smooth.*

Or a 40-30-30 Nutrition Bar	1 bar	1 bar	1 bar	1 bar

DINNER	A	B	C	D
Ground Turkey Burger				
Ground Turkey Breast Patty	3 oz.	3.5 oz.	4 oz.	4 oz.
Onion, chopped	1/2 c.	1/2 c.	1/2 c.	1/2 c.
Red Pepper, chopped	1/2 c.	1/2 c.	1/2 c.	1/2 c.
Mushrooms, chopped	1/2 c.	1/2 c.	1/2 c.	1/2 c.
Broccoli, spears	1 c.	1 1/2 c.	1 1/2 c.	1 1/2 c.
Applesauce, unsweetened	1/2 c.	2/3 c.	1 c.	1 c.
Green Salad	1	1	1	1
Salad Dressing, full-fat, your choice	2 t.	2 t.	1 T.	1 T.

Directions: *Grill ground turkey patty. Saute onion, red pepper, and mushrooms in 1 t. whipped butter and serve over turkey patty. Serve with steamed broccoli, applesauce, and green salad with salad dressing.*

■ Beverages: Always consume an 8 oz. appropriate beverage with each meal (see Chapter 9).

■ Nutrition bar: A 40-30-30 Nutrition Bar may be substituted for breakfast, lunch, or snack when desired.

**F
A
T

F
L
U
S
H**

MEALS

FBN Fat-Flush Meals—Example Day 6

AMOUNT FOR MEAL PLANNERS

BREAKFAST	A	B	C	D
Turkey Sausage and Fruit				
Turkey Sausage, low-fat	2.5 oz.	2.5 oz.	4 oz.	6 oz.
Orange, sliced	1 large	1 large	2 med.	2 med.

Directions: *Serve fried turkey sausage with fresh sliced oranges.*

LUNCH	A	B	C	D
Chili and Fruit				
No-Bean Chili* (see recipe)	1 c.	1 1/2 c.	1 1/2 c.	2 c.
Apple, small	1	1	1	1

Directions: *Have chili with an apple.*

* No-Bean Chili recipe: 1 lb. lean ground turkey breast, browned in 2 T. safflower oil. Add 1/2 c. chopped celery, 1 c. chopped green pepper, 1 c. chopped onion, 1 c. chopped mushrooms, and 1/2 c. chopped fresh parsley. Add 1 package of chili seasoning along with one 14.5 oz. can tomatoes with juice, diced, one 15 oz. tomato sauce and one 8 oz. can of tomato puree. Cook for at least one hour or longer. Makes approximately 8 cups. If you like your chili spicy, add 1/2-1 t. crushed red pepper flakes.

SNACK	A	B	C	D
Plain, Low-Fat Yogurt				
Plain, Low-Fat Yogurt	1	1	1	1
Or a 40-30-30 Nutrition Bar	**1 bar**	**1 bar**	**1 bar**	**1 bar**

DINNER	A	B	C	D
Teriyaki Chicken Kabobs				
Chicken Breast, cubed	3 oz.	4 oz.	5 oz.	5 oz.
Teriyaki Marinade*	1 T.	1 1/2 T.	2 T.	2 T.
Green Bell Pepper, cubed	1/2	1	1	1
Onion, sweet, cubed	1/2	3/4	1	1
Cherry Tomatoes	4	6	6	6
Pineapple Chunks	3/4 c.	3/4 c.	1 c.	1 c.
Green Salad	1 c.	1 c.	1 c.	1 c.
Salad Dressing, full-fat, your choice	2 t.	1 T.	1 1/2 T.	1 1/2 T.

Directions: *On several skewers, alternate marinated chicken, green bell peppers, onion, cherry tomatoes and pineapple chunks. Grill or broil and baste with any remaining marinade and pineapple juice. Serve with salad and a full-fat salad dressing of your choice.*

* Teriyaki Marinade recipe: Combine 2 T. vegetable oil, 2 T. soy sauce, 2 t. brown sugar, 1/2 t. garlic powder and 1/2 T. sherry. Add chicken and marinate for several hours. (You may substitute with 2 1/2 T. of bottled Teriyaki marinade).

■ Beverages: Always consume an 8 oz. appropriate beverage with each meal (see Chapter 9).

■ Nutrition bar: A 40-30-30 Nutrition Bar may be substituted for breakfast, lunch, or snack when desired.

FAT FLUSH

MEALS

FBN Fat-Flush Meals—Example Day 7

AMOUNT FOR MEAL PLANNERS

BREAKFAST	A	B	C	D
Sliced Ham and Fruit Plate				
Ham, breakfast, sliced	3 oz.	3 oz.	5 oz.	7 oz.
Grapefruit, half	1	1	1	2
Apple, sliced	1/2	1/2	1	1

Directions: *Heat breakfast ham and serve with grapefruit and sliced apple.*

LUNCH	A	B	C	D
Cantaloupe Fruit Salad				
Cantaloupe, 1/2 of a 5" melon	1	1	1	1
Cottage Cheese, 2% low-fat	2/3 c.	1 c.	1 c.	1 1/2 c.
Grapes, green or red, seedless	-	5	5	10
Strawberries, sliced	1/4 c.	1/2 c.	1/2 c.	1 c.
Sunflower Seeds, raw	1 t.	2 t.	2 t.	1 T.

Directions: *Hollow out cantaloupe. Fill with cottage cheese and top with cubed cantaloupe, sliced grapes and strawberries. Sprinkle with sunflower seeds.*

SNACK	A	B	C	D
Turkey and Fruit				
Turkey, sliced thin	2 oz.	2 oz.	2 oz.	2 oz.
Apple, medium	1	1	1	1

Directions: *Have sliced turkey with apple.*

Or a 40-30-30 Nutrition Bar	**1 bar**	**1 bar**	**1 bar**	**1 bar**

DINNER	A	B	C	D
Grilled Pork Tenderloin and Applesauce				
Grilled Pork Tenderloin, lean	3.5 oz.	4 oz.	4.5 oz.	4.5 oz.
Broccoli	1 c.	1 c.	1 1/2 c.	1 1/2 c.
Applesauce	1/2 c.	3/4 c.	1 c.	1 c.
Spinach, cleaned, dried and torn	2 c.	2 c.	3 c.	3 c.
Mandarin Orange Slices, water packed, drained	1/4 c.	1/4 c.	1/4 c.	1/4 c.
Salad Dressing* (see recipe)	1 T.	1 T.	1 1/2 T.	1 1/2 T.
Almonds, raw	1 t.	1 t.	1 t.	1 t.

Directions: *Season pork tenderloin with garlic, salt, and pepper and grill or bake in foil. Serve with steamed broccoli spears, applesauce, and spinach salad.*

* Spinach Salad recipe: Toss spinach, mandarin oranges, almonds, and dressing. Dressing: 1 T. vegetable oil, 2 t. red wine vinegar, 1 t. cider vinegar, 1/4 t. sugar or crystalline fructose, and a sprinkle of garlic salt, and pepper.

■ Beverages: Always consume an 8 oz. appropriate beverage with each meal (see Chapter 9).

■ Nutrition bar: A 40-30-30 Nutrition Bar may be substituted for breakfast, lunch, or snack when desired.

FAT FLUSH MEALS

FBN VEGETARIAN MEALS

FBN Vegetarian Meals have been designed with a variety of high- and low-glycemic carbohydrate and quality protein and fat. They contain no animal protein except eggs and dairy sources (ovolacto vegetarian). We chose to include eggs and dairy to ensure adequate amounts of quality protein providing a high ratio of the essential amino acids. For strict vegans, simply replace any objectional protein with equal amounts of tofu or tempeh.

If you are not a vegetarian, you can still use any of the delicious meals we have included in this section. They contain sample meals that follow *40-30-30 Fat-Burning Nutrition*, and are suitable for everyone. We also include the use of a 40-30-30 Nutrition bar as a meal replacement or snack.

Begin by following the meals we have provided. Once you get the hang of it, you can design your own meals using the *40-30-30 Fat-Burning Nutrition* ratio with your favorite foods and recipes. Our goal is to provide you with sample meal planners that are perfectly balanced and provide adequate macronutrients for your unique requirements.

V
E
G
E
T
A
R
I
A
N

MEALS

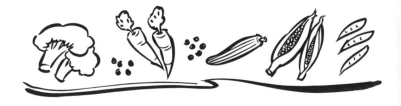

FBN Vegetarian Meals—Example Day 1

AMOUNTS FOR MEAL PLANNERS

BREAKFAST	A	B	C	D
Boca Burger Breakfast Sandwich				
Boca Burger	1	1	1 1/2	2
Pita Pocket, whole wheat	3/4	3/4	1	1 1/2
Lettuce, red leaf, shredded	1/4 c.	1/4 c.	1/4 c.	1/4 c.
Tomato Slice	1	1	2	2
Mayonnaise, safflower	1 t.	1 t.	2 t.	1 T.

Directions: *Place Boca burger, hot or cold, in pita pocket with lettuce, tomato, and mayonnaise.*

LUNCH	A	B	C	D
Cottage Cheese and Fruit				
Cottage Cheese, 2% low-fat	2/3 c.	1 c.	1 c.	1 1/3 c.
Orange	1 small	1 medium	1 medium	1 large
Bagel, whole wheat	1/2	1/2	1/2	3/4

Directions: *Have cottage cheese with fresh orange and bagel.*

SNACK	A	B	C	D
Fruit Protein Shake				
Whey Protein Powder				
(1 scoop = 16 g)	1	1	1	1
Banana, frozen	1/3	1/3	1/3	1/3
Peaches, frozen, unsweetened	1 c.	1 c.	1 c.	1 c.
Almonds, raw	2 t.	2 t.	2 t.	2 t.
Water	1/2 c.	1/2 c.	1/2 c.	1/2 c.

Directions: *Combine all ingredients in a high-speed blender and blend till smooth.*

Or a 40-30-30 Nutrition Bar	**1 bar**	**1 bar**	**1 bar**	**1 bar**

DINNER	A	B	C	D
Vegetarian Chili				
Vegetarian Chili * (see recipe)	1 1/3 c.	1 1/2 c.	2 c.	2 c.
Green Salad	1 c.	2 c.	2 c.	2 c.
Salad Dressing, full-fat, your choice	2 t.	2 t.	1 T.	1 T.

Directions: *Have a bowl of chili with a dinner salad with a full-fat salad dressing of your choice.*

* Vegetarian Chili Recipe: Brown 1 1/2 pounds of diced extra high protein, low fat soy tempeh, in 1 T. safflower oil. Add 1/2 c. chopped celery, 1 c. chopped green pepper, 1 c. chopped onion, 1/2 c. fresh parsley, and 1 c. chopped mushrooms. Stir in 1 package chili seasonings. Add 14.5 oz. canned tomatoes with juice, 15 oz. canned tomato sauce, an 8 oz. can of tomato puree and a 15 oz. can of black beans. Mix well and simmer for at least one hour or more, or make it a day ahead and reheat. Smaller servings are great for lunch. If you like your chili spicy, add 1/2-1 t. crushed red pepper flakes.

■ Beverages: Always consume an 8 oz. appropriate beverage with each meal (see Chapter 9).

■ Nutrition bar: A 40-30-30 Nutrition Bar may be substituted for breakfast, lunch, or snack when desired.

V E G E T A R I A N

MEALS

FBN Vegetarian Meals—Example Day 2

AMOUNTS FOR MEAL PLANNERS

BREAKFAST	A	B	C	D
Peanut Butter and Banana Protein Shake				
Whey Protein Powder				
(1 scoop = 16 g)	3/4	3/4	1	1 1/4
Peanut Butter, all natural	2 t.	2 t.	1 T.	1 1/2 T.
Banana, frozen	1/3	1/3	1/2	1
Milk, non-fat	1/2 c.	1/2 c.	1/2 c.	3/4 c.

Directions: *Combine all ingredients in a high-speed blender and blend till smooth.*

LUNCH	A	B	C	D
Boca Burger				
Boca Burger Patty	1	1 1/2	1 1/2	2
Hamburger Bun, whole wheat	1	1	1	2
Lettuce, leaf	1	1	1	2
Tomato, slice	1	1	1	2
Catsup	1 t.	2 t.	2 t.	1 T.

Directions: *Heat Boca burger patty and place on hamburger bun with lettuce, tomato slice and catsup.*

SNACK	A	B	C	D
String Cheese and Fruit				
String Cheese, reduced fat, 1 oz.	1	1	1	1
Grapes, red or green, seedless	15	15	15	15

Directions: *Have cheese with fruit.*

Or a 40-30-30 Nutrition Bar	**1 bar**	**1 bar**	**1 bar**	**1 bar**

DINNER	A	B	C	D
Tofu Fried Rice				
Tofu, low-fat	1/2 c.	2/3 c.	3/4 c.	3/4 c.
Vegetable Oil, safflower	1 t.	2 t.	2 T.	1 T.
Carrots, Onions, Red Pepper,				
Broccoli, and Mushrooms, diced	3/4 c.	1 c.	1 c.	1 c.
Soy Sauce, to taste				
Pepper, to taste				
Rice, brown, cooked	2/3 c.	3/4 c.	1 c.	1 c.
Green Salad	1 c.	2 c.	2 c.	2 c.
Salad Dressing, non-fat	1 T.	1 T.	1 T.	1 T.

Directions: *Heat oil in heavy skillet or wok. Brown tofu. Add vegetables till tender. Add cooked brown rice and season to taste with soy sauce and pepper. Serve with green salad and non-fat salad dressing.*

■ Beverages: Always consume an 8 oz. appropriate beverage with each meal (see Chapter 9).

■ Nutrition bar: A 40-30-30 Nutrition Bar may be substituted for breakfast, lunch, or snack when desired.

**V
E
G
E
T
A
R
I
A
N**

MEALS

FBN Vegetarian Meals—Example Day 3

AMOUNTS FOR MEAL PLANNERS

BREAKFAST	A	B	C	D
Scrambled Eggs				
Egg, whole	1	1	2	3
Egg Whites	2	2	3	4
Toast, whole grain	1	1	2	2
Grapefruit, half	1	1	1	2

Directions: *Scramble eggs and serve with toast and grapefruit.*

LUNCH	A	B	C	D
Berry Yogurt Protein Shake				
Whey Protein Powder				
(1 scoop = 16 g)	1	1 1/2	1 1/2	2
Yogurt, fat-free with fruit	4 oz.	6 oz.	6 oz.	8 oz.
Blueberries, frozen, unsweetened	1/3 c.	1/3 c.	1/3 c.	1/3 c.
Water	1/2 c.	1/2 c.	1/2 c.	1/2 c.
Almonds, raw	2 t.	1 1/2 T.	1 1/2 T.	2 T.

Directions: *Combine all ingredients in a high-speed blender and blend till smooth.*

SNACK	A	B	C	D
Cottage Cheese with Pineapple				
Cottage Cheese with Pineapple,				
low fat, 4 oz.	1	1	1	1

Directions: *Buy prepared low-fat cottage cheese with pineapple added.*

Or a 40-30-30 Nutrition Bar	**1 bar**	**1 bar**	**1 bar**	**1 bar**

DINNER	A	B	C	D
Teriyaki Boca Burgers and Vegetables				
Boca Burger Patty	2	2	2 1/2	2 1/2
Teriyaki Sauce	1 T	1 T.	2 T.	2 T.
Sauted Vegetables:				
Onion	1/2 c.	1/2 c.	1/2 c.	1/2 c.
Zucchini	1 c.	1 c.	1 c.	1 c.
Yam, baked	1/4 c.	1/2 c.	3/4 c.	3/4 c.
Green Salad	1 c.	1 c.	2 c.	2 c.
Salad Dressing, full-fat, your choice	2 t.	2 t.	1 T.	1 T.

Directions: *Grill Boca burger, baste with teriyaki marinade. Saute sliced onions and zucchini in 1 t. safflower oil. Bake or microwave yam till tender. Serve with a green salad and salad dressing.*

■ Beverages: Always consume an 8 oz. appropriate beverage with each meal (see Chapter 9).

■ Nutrition bar: A 40-30-30 Nutrition Bar may be substituted for breakfast, lunch, or snack when desired.

V
E
G
E
T
A
R
I
A
N

MEALS

FBN Vegetarian Meals—Example Day 4

AMOUNTS FOR MEAL PLANNERS

BREAKFAST	A	B	C	D
Yogurt Cheese				
Yogurt, vanilla, low-fat	1/2 c.	1/2 c.	1 c.	1 1/3 c.
Cottage Cheese, 2% low-fat	1/3 c.	1/3 c.	1/2 c.	3/4 c.
Almonds, raw	1 t.	1 t.	2 t.	1 T.

Directions: *Combine yogurt with cottage cheese and top with almonds.*
Note: If using fat-free yogurt or cottage cheese, increase almonds.

LUNCH	A	B	C	D
Grilled Cheese Sandwich				
Bread, oat bran, reduced-calorie	2	3	3	4
Cheese, non-fat, 1 oz. slices	2	2	2	4
Cheese, 1/3 less fat, 1 oz. slices	1	2	2	2
Olive Oil	1 t.	1 1/2 t.	1 1/2 t.	2 t.
Tomato Slice	1	2	2	2
Pickle Spear, dill	1	1	1	1
Carrot Sticks	4	4	4	4
Cucumber Rounds	1/2 c.	1/2 c.	1/2 c.	1/2 c.

Directions: *Lightly brush olive oil on one side of the bread. Layer cheese slices and grill oiled sides of bread under broiler or brown in a skillet. Add tomato slice and pickle or serve them on the side. Have with crisp carrot sticks and cucumber rounds.*

SNACK	A	B	C	D
Hard Boiled Eggs and Fruit				
Egg, whole	1	1	1	1
Egg Whites	2	2	2	2
Apple, small	1	1	1	1

Directions: *Peel three hard boiled eggs and discard two yolks. Have with apple.*

Or a 40-30-30 Nutrition Bar	1 bar	1 bar	1 bar	1 bar

DINNER	A	B	C	D
Tempeh Stir-Fry				
Garlic, one clove, minced	1	1	1	1
Ginger, ground	1/2 t.	1/2 t.	1/2 t.	1/2 t.
Vegetable Oil	2 t.	2 t.	1 T.	1 T.
Tempeh, low-fat, cubed	4 oz.	4.5 oz.	5 oz.	5 oz.
Snow Peas, whole	1/4 c.	1/4 c.	1/2 c.	1/2 c.
Red Bell Pepper, strips	1/4 c.	1/4 c.	1/2 c.	1/2 c.
Green Onions, sliced	2	2	3	3
Broccoli, sliced	1/4 c.	1/4 c.	1/2 c.	1/2 c.
Carrot, thinly sliced	1/4 c.	1/4 c.	1/2 c.	1/2 c.
Brown Rice, cooked	1/2 c.	2/3 c.	3/4 c.	3/4 c.

Directions: *In a large skillet or wok, heat oil. Add garlic and ginger for 30 seconds. Add tempeh and stir-fry for 3 minutes. Add vegetables and stir-fry until crisp-tender, about 5 minutes. Add 1/4 c. orange juice and 1 t. soy sauce. Serve over brown rice.*

■ Beverages: Always consume an 8 oz. appropriate beverage with each meal (see Chapter 9).

■ Nutrition bar: A 40-30-30 Nutrition Bar may be substituted for breakfast, lunch, or snack when desired.

V
E
G
E
T
A
R
I
A
N

MEALS

FBN Vegetarian Meals—Example Day 5

AMOUNTS FOR MEAL PLANNERS

BREAKFAST	A	B	C	D
Tempeh Breakfast Burrito				
Tortilla, flour, 7"	1	1	1 1/2	2
Tempeh, crumbled	3 oz.	3 oz.	4.5 oz.	6 oz.
Salsa	2 T.	2 T.	3 T.	4 T.

Directions: *Stir fry tempeh in salsa till hot, serve in a warmed tortilla.*

LUNCH	A	B	C	D
Egg Salad Sandwich				
Egg, whole	1	2	2	2
Egg Whites	2	3	3	5
Pickle Relish, sweet	1 T.	2 T.	2 T.	2 T.
Celery, diced	1 T.	2 T.	2 T.	2 T.
Mayonnaise, reduced-fat	2 t.	2 T.	2 T.	2 1/2 T.
Mustard, prepared	1 t.	2 t.	2 t.	2 t.
Bread, whole grain	2 *	2	2	3
Tangerine	1/2	1	1	1

Directions: *Hard boil eggs. Cool, peel and discard some yolks. Dice and mix with pickles, celery, mayonnaise and mustard. Spread on bread and serve with a tangerine or other small fruit.*

SNACK	A	B	C	D
Plain, Low-Fat Yogurt				
Plain, Low-Fat Yogurt	1	1	1	1
Or a 40-30-30 Nutrition Bar	**1 bar**	**1 bar**	**1 bar**	**1 bar**

DINNER	A	B	C	D
Cottage Cheese and Fruit Plate				
Cottage Cheese, 2% low fat	1 c.	1 1/4 c.	1 1/2 c.	1 1/2 c.
Cantaloupe	1/2	1/2	1/2	1/2
Strawberries	1/2 c.	2/3 c.	1 c.	1 c.
Grapes, red or green, seedless	5	10	10	10
Banana, medium	1/3	1/3	1/2	1/2

Directions: *Using melon baller, scoop out flesh from half a cantaloupe into balls. Combine with sliced strawberries, grapes, and bananas. Place cottage cheese in hollowed out melon half and top with all of the fruit.*

* Reduced Calorie

■ Beverages: Always consume an 8 oz. appropriate beverage with each meal (see Chapter 9).

■ Nutrition bar: A 40-30-30 Nutrition Bar may be substituted for breakfast, lunch, or snack when desired.

VEGETARIAN

MEALS

FBN Vegetarian Meals—Example Day 6

AMOUNTS FOR MEAL PLANNERS

BREAKFAST	A	B	C	D
Oatmeal and Cottage Cheese				
Oatmeal, cooked in water	1/2 c.	1/2 c.	3/4 c.	1 c.
Cottage Cheese, 2% low-fat	1/2 c.	1/2 c.	3/4 c.	1 c.
Applesauce, unsweetened	2 T.	2 T.	1/4 c.	1/2 c.
Cinnamon	sprinkle	sprinkle	sprinkle	sprinkle
Almonds, raw	1 t.	1 t.	1 T.	1 1/2 T.

Directions: *Cook oatmeal in water as directed. Add applesauce, cinnamon, and almonds. Serve cottage cheese on the side or mix with cooked oatmeal.*

LUNCH	A	B	C	D
Tofu Fried Rice				
Tofu, low-fat	4 oz.	6 oz.	6 oz.	7.5 oz.
Broccoli, diced	1/2 c.	1/2 c.	1/2 c.	1 c.
Soy Sauce, reduced sodium	2 t.	1 T.	1 T.	1 1/2 T.
Vegetable Oil, safflower	1 t.	2 t.	2 t.	2 t.
Brown Rice, cooked	1/2 c.	2/3 c.	2/3 c.	1 c.

Directions: *Heat vegetable oil in skillet or wok and add tofu till browned. Add broccoli and soy sauce and stir-fry 4-5 minutes. Add cooked rice and fry till done.*

SNACK	A	B	C	D
Peanut Butter Shake				
Whey Protein Powder				
(1 scoop = 16 g)	1	1	1	1
Banana, frozen, medium	1/2	1/2	1/2	1/2
Peanut Butter, all natural	2 t.	2 t.	2 t.	2 t.
Water	1/2 c.	1/2 c.	1/2 c.	1/2 c.

Directions: *Combine all ingredients in a high-speed blender and blend till smooth.*

Or a 40-30-30 Nutrition Bar	**1 bar**	**1 bar**	**1 bar**	**1 bar**

DINNER	A	B	C	D
Cheese Omelette				
Egg, whole	1	2	2	2
Egg Whites	3	3	4	4
Cheese, Swiss, Alpine Lace Lite	1 oz.	1 oz.	1 1/4 oz.	1 1/4 oz.
Spinach, cleaned, dried,				
and chopped	5	5	5	5
Potatoes, new, 1 1/2" diameter	3	4	5	5
Green Salad	1 c.	1 c.	2 c.	2 c.
Salad Dressing, non-fat	1 T.	1 T.	1 T.	1 T.

Directions: *Scramble eggs. Pour into hot non-stick omelette pan, add cheese and chopped spinach leaves to make omelette. Serve with sliced new potatoes and a green salad with non-fat salad dressing.*

■ Beverages: Always consume an 8 oz. appropriate beverage with each meal (see Chapter 9).

■ Nutrition bar: A 40-30-30 Nutrition Bar may be substituted for breakfast, lunch, or snack when desired.

FBN Vegetarian Meals—Example Day 7

AMOUNTS FOR MEAL PLANNERS

BREAKFAST	A	B	C	D
Cereal and Soy Milk				
Shredded Wheat Cereal (spoon size)	1/3 c.	1/3 c.	2/3 c.	1 c.
Soy Milk, unsweetened	6 oz.	6 oz.	8 oz.	8 oz.
Soy Protein Powder	1/2 oz.	1/2 oz.	1 oz.	1 1/2 oz.
Orange, medium size	1/2	1/2	1	1 1/2

Directions: *Blend soy milk and soy protein powder, pour over cereal and serve with a fresh orange.*

LUNCH	A	B	C	D
Tempeh Caesar Salad				
Tempeh, pre-cooked and cooled	3 oz.	4 oz.	4 oz.	5 oz.
Romaine Lettuce, cleaned, dried, and torn	3 c.	3 c.	3 c.	4 c.
Parmesan Cheese, finely grated	1 t.	1 t.	1 t.	1 t.
Croutons, low-fat	1/2 oz.	1 oz.	1 oz.	1 1/2 oz.
Caesar Salad Dressing, bottled or recipe*	1 T.	1 T.	1 T.	2 T.

Directions: *Pre-cook and cool tempeh. Clean, dry, and tear romaine lettuce. Add tempeh, toss with Caesar salad dressing and top with croutons and parmesan cheese. Add black pepper to taste.*

* Caesar salad dressing recipe: 1 T. olive oil, 1 T. red wine vinegar, 1/2 T. lemon juice, 1 small clove of garlic, pressed or 1/8 t. garlic powder, 1/2 t. Worcestershire sauce, 1/2 t. anchovy paste, 1/2 t. dry mustard, 1/2 t. fresh ground pepper, 1/8 t. salt (optional). Place all ingredients in a small jar and shake till blended.

SNACK	A	B	C	D
Cheese and Crackers				
String Cheese, low-fat, 1 oz.	1	1	1	1
Rye Crackers (Rykrisp)	2	2	2	2
Directions: *Have string cheese with rye crackers.*				
Or a 40-30-30 Nutrition Bar	**1 bar**	**1 bar**	**1 bar**	**1 bar**

DINNER	A	B	C	D
Spaghetti with Tempeh Pasta Sauce				
Spaghetti, cooked	2/3 c.	2/3 c.	3/4 c.	3/4 c.
Tempeh, crumbled	3 oz.	4 oz.	6 oz.	6 oz.
Pasta Sauce, fat- and sugar-free	1/2 c.	1/2 c.	1/2 c.	1/2 c.
Asparagus, spears	4	6	6	6
Green Salad	1 c.	2 c.	2 c.	2 c.
Salad Dressing, Italian, full-fat	2 t.	1 T.	1 T.	1 T.

Directions: *Cook crumbled tempeh in skillet till browned. Add pasta sauce till hot and serve over cooked spaghetti. Serve with steamed asparagus spears and a green salad with Italian salad dressing.*

■ Beverages: Always consume an 8 oz. appropriate beverage with each meal (see Chapter 9).

■ Nutrition bar: A 40-30-30 Nutrition Bar may be substituted for breakfast, lunch, or snack when desired.

V
E
G
E
T
A
R
I
A
N

MEALS

Chapter 9

MAKE WATER YOUR FIRST PRIORITY

Your body requires a *minimum* of 2-4 quarts of water each day. Because of the high amounts of water contained in the fruits and vegetables recommended in *40-30-30 Fat-Burning Nutrition*, you will be getting a lot of the water you need from foods. However, additional water is vital for good health and to maximize the fat burning process.

Listed below are several recommendations for appropriate *40-30-30 Fat-Burning Nutrition* beverages:

☑ Always start your day with an 8 oz. glass of water.

☑ Try to consume *at least* four to six 8 oz. glasses of water each day.

☑ If you exercise a lot, have a strenuous job, or live in a hot climate, you may need to double the recommended water intake.

☑ *40-30-30 Fat-Burning Nutrition* recommended beverages include water, mineral water, decaffeinated coffee and tea, herbal teas, and caffeine-free drinks. Since sugar can cause a rapid rise in blood sugar levels and stimulate insulin release, it is best to avoid sugar-containing drinks of any kind.

☑ In general, we recommend that you avoid fruit juices or consume them in very small, diluted amounts (2-3 oz.), and have them as part of your regular meal. Dilute canned juices and concentrates with twice as much or more water than recommended. If juicing, minimize high-glycemic fruit, carrot and beet juices and increase the lower-glycemic, highly nutritious green and red vegetable juices like broccoli, cabbage, celery, parsley, and spinach.

☑ Caffeine can also stimulate the production of insulin, so avoid or minimize caffeine-containing beverages. Switch to decaffeinated beverages or a mix of half regular and half decaffeinated. Try herbal tea or hot water with lemon instead of coffee.

NOTE: If you are currently using large amounts of caffeine-containing beverages, gradually reduce their consumption to eliminate headaches and energy slumps that can result from caffeine withdrawal. <u>Do not stop them all at once</u>!

• One of our favorite beverages is a low-fat decaffeinated latté, hot or iced. The milk is perfectly balanced with 1/3 more carbohydrate than protein.

• If you don't have trouble digesting milk, low-fat and non-fat milk has a perfect 1.3 to 1 ratio of carbohydrate to protein. When drinking milk with a meal, be sure to include it as part of the carbohydrate, protein, and fat of that meal.

• When drinking an alcoholic beverage, have it with a high protein appetizer or with your meal. Alcohol converts into sugar once consumed, so limit your consumption for best results.

Chapter 10

Have more carbohydrate than protein. Remember to always have approximately one-third more carbohydrate than protein at each meal (a 1.3 to 1 ratio of carbohydrate to protein), and choose low-fat, high-quality protein every time you eat. You don't want to have only carbohydrate for breakfast and protein at lunch. It will not work. A hormonal response is triggered every time you eat a meal or snack. Each meal should contain the proper *40-30-30 Fat-Burning Nutrition* ratio to stabilize blood sugar levels, control insulin, and elevate glucagon, the fat mobilization hormone.

Follow the plan most suited for you. Follow the recommended amount for your personal requirements found in the Sample Meal Planners. You need to eat adequate amounts of carbohydrate, protein, and fat at each meal to maximize fat burning. Skipping meals or reducing the amount of your food intake will <u>not</u> result in accelerating the fat burning process.

Balance your blood sugar. When blood sugar is balanced, not only will you lose unwanted body fat, but you will experience increased levels of physical and mental energy, improved tissue repair and recovery from exercise, and maintain or increase lean body mass (muscle). You should also notice a lack of hunger between meals, fewer sugar cravings, less fatigue, less lightheadedness, and fewer mood swings.

Have your body fat analyzed. Body fat testing is the most effective method of monitoring the ratio of fat loss to muscle loss. If you can, have your body fat analyzed and have it rechecked every 4-6 weeks. Your doctor and most health clubs can analyze your percentage of body fat. When retesting, always use the same method you originally used and, if possible, have the same person with the same machine retest you.

Total your inches lost to monitor your success. The scale is not the most effective way to determine your success with *40-30-30 Fat-Burning Nutrition*. Since one pound of fat is much larger in size than one pound of muscle (muscle weight is very dense), determine your success by the way your clothes fit. We also suggest using a tape measure to monitor the inches you are losing. If measuring only one body part, test your waist.

Follow your plan. It may take 2-3 weeks to get your body to maximize the fat burning process, so stick with it. If you have been a "carbo junkie," it may take even longer for your body to adjust and to start burning fat efficiently. We have seen unbelievable results with *40-30-30 Fat-Burning Nutrition* after about the third week. And we have never seen it fail. Some people just do not follow the program or will not stop over-eating carbohydrate, but for those that do, *40-30-30 Fat-Burning Nutrition* works!

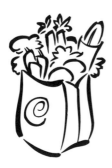

Eat protein before eating carbohydrates. To maximize the stimulation of the fat-burning hormone glucagon, eat a bite or two of protein *first*, before eating any carbohydrates. This will help slow the digestion and absorption of the carbohydrate in that meal resulting in better stabilization of blood sugar levels.

Eat raw almonds and walnuts. Raw almonds and walnuts are some of the best sources of "good fats." Try adding one teaspoon of raw nuts to salads, protein drinks, cereals, cottage cheese, and so forth when fat is too low in a meal.

Don't overcook rice and pasta. Undercooking rice and pasta (al dente) will lower their glycemic index value. This will slow their digestion to help stabilize blood sugar levels and to minimize the release of the fat-storage hormone, insulin.

Limit starches to one serving per meal. If you have potatoes, rice, or pasta at dinner, don't have bread too. Also, avoid starchy vegetables like corn or peas in that meal and choose a low glycemic vegetable like asparagus, broccoli, or green beans instead. For fastest fat loss, avoid all starchy, high-glycemic carbohydrates at dinner and eat plenty of fruits and vegetables as your main source of carbohydrate. (See the *40-30-30 FBN Fat-Flush Meals* in Chapter 8, *"Putting It All Together"*). Limit or avoid starches and sugars after 7:00 p.m.

High-sugar carbohydrates and very high-glycemic carbohydrates like popcorn eaten prior to bed can easily elevate blood sugar levels, stimulate insulin, and block the release of human growth hormone. It is especially important not to have sweets or very high-glycemic carbohydrate within two hours before bed. The glucose you don't burn off will be stored as fat.

Limit starches when dessert is included in the meal. When occasionally having dessert with dinner, limit or avoid all starches like potatoes, rice, pasta, and bread, and increase the vegetables and fruits in the meal. Eat only a portion of the dessert and count it as the major portion of carbohydrate in that meal.

Consume alcoholic beverages with protein foods. If you have an alcoholic beverage, control the elevation of blood sugar it can cause by having it with your meal or with a high-protein appetizer.

Have lots of fluids daily. Drink 6 to 8 glasses of water or appropriate beverages each day. (See Chapter 9,"*40-30-30 Fat-Burning Nutrition Recommended Beverages*").

Exercise. Exercise speeds up the fat-burning process by burning calories, increasing the metabolic rate, and lowering insulin levels. When insulin is lowered, glucagon is elevated, and exercise really starts to pay off by burning maximum levels of stored body fat for energy. Exercise also releases human growth hormone (HGH), another powerful fat-burning hormone. The type and amount of exercise you choose is up to you. We highly recommend that you exercise a minimum of three times per week for 30 minutes each session. Be sure to include both aerobic *and* strength training for the most effective hormonal response.

> We highly recommend that you exercise a minimum of three times per week for 30 minutes each session.

Don't worry if you get off track. This is not a diet, but a program of learning how to maximize your hormonal response with foods *every time you eat*! If you get off track, simply restart the fat burning process at your next meal.

Food Value Guide

Listed below are commonly used foods. Included are the macronutrient values of the foods and a rating of the glycemic index level for carbohydrate. The foods listed are some of the best sources to be used with *40-30-30 Fat-Burning Nutrition*.

Protein Sources (Low-Fat)   Macronutrients

FOOD	SERVING SIZE	PROTEIN GRAMS	CARB. GRAMS	FAT GRAMS
Beef				
Beef brisket, X-lean	4 oz.	35	0	11
Beef chuck, X-lean	4 oz.	37	0	9
Lean flank steak	4 oz.	31	0	11
Ground sirloin, X-lean	4 oz.	30	0	9
Chicken				
Breast, w/o skin, roasted	4 oz.	35	0	4
Light meat, w/o skin, roasted	4 oz.	35	0	5
Dark meat, w/o skin, roasted	4 oz.	31	0	11
Dairy				
Cheese				
Colby, low-fat	1 oz.	4	1	2
Cheddar, lite	1 oz.	6	2	4
Cheddar, fat-free	1 oz.	8	1	0
American, lite	1 oz.	6	2	4
American, fat-free	1 oz.	8	1	0
Mozzarella, lite	1 oz.	9	1	2
Mozzarella, fat-free	1 oz.	9	0	0
Parmesan, grated, lite	1 Tbs.	2	.2	1.5
Provolone, lite	1 oz.	8	1	4
Ricotta, lite	1 oz.	4	1	2
String cheese, lite	1 oz.	9	1	2
Swiss, lite	1 oz.	8	1	6
Swiss, fat-free	1 oz.	8	1	0
Cottage cheese 2%	1 c.	28	8	4
Cottage cheese 1%	1 c.	28	8	2
Cottage cheese, non-fat	1 c.	28	8	0
Cottage cheese, dry curd	1/2 cup	16	6	0
Cream cheese, non-fat	1 oz.	4	3	0
Milk, 2% low-fat	8 oz.	8	12	5
Milk, 2% low-fat, protein fort.	8 oz.	10	14	5
Milk, 1% low-fat	8 oz.	8	12	3
Milk, 1% low-fat, protein fort.	8 oz.	10	14	2
Milk, skim	8 oz.	9	12	0
Milk, skim, protein fortified	8 oz.	10	14	1
Sour cream, non-fat	2 Tbsp.	3	1	0
Yogurt, plain, fat-free	8 oz.	13	17	0
Yogurt, plain, low-fat	8 oz.	12	16	3
Yoplait Light	6 oz.	6	13	0
Knudsen Cal 70	6 oz.	6	11	0
Deer/Venison, roasted without skin	4 oz.	34	0	4

FOOD	SERVING SIZE	PROTEIN GRAMS	CARB. GRAMS	FAT GRAMS
Eggs				
Large whole egg	one	6	0	5
Egg white	one	4	0	0
Egg yolk	one	3	0	5
Egg substitute, liquid	1/2 cup	15	0	4
Egg substitute, frozen	1/2 cup			
Lamb				
Leg, shank, lean only	4 oz.	32	0	8
Sirloin, lean only	4 oz.	32	0	10
Pork				
Ham, extra-lean, (5%) sliced	5 oz.	30	2	8
Pork tenderloin, roasted	4 oz.	36	0	5
Protein Powder				
Whey Protein Powder	1 scoop	16	2	1
Seafood				
Bass, freshwater	6 oz.	28	0	0
Bass, striped	5 oz.	30	0	4
Carp	6 oz.	30	0	10
Clams, raw	1/2 cup	29	6	2
Catfish, channel	6 oz.	30	0	7
Cod, Atlantic (cooked)	5 oz.	32	0	1
Crab, Alaskan King (imitation)	7 oz.	23	20	3
Crab, Alaskan King (raw)	6 oz.	32	0	1
Crayfish	5 oz.	33	0	2
Flounder	6 oz.	32	0	2
Haddock	6 oz.	28	0	0
Halibut	5 oz.	37	0	4
Lobster	6 oz.	32	1	2
Monkfish	6 oz.	31	0	3
Mussels	5 oz.	33	10	6
Oysters, raw	one	5	3	1
Perch, Ocean	5 oz.	33	0	3
Salmon, smoked	6 oz.	31	0	9
Salmon, Coho	4 oz.	30	0	9
Scallops	12 large	30	4	1
Sea bass	5 oz.	33	0	4
Shrimp	5 oz.	30	0	2
Snapper	5 oz.	29	0	2
Sole	7 oz.	29	0	1
Swordfish	6 oz.	33	0	7
Rainbow trout	6 oz.	34	0	6
Tuna, blue fin	5 oz.	33	0	7
Tuna, albacore, canned	4 oz.	30	0	2
Tuna, yellow fin	4 oz.	33	0	1
Turkey				
Breast, w/o skin, roasted	4 oz.	34	0	1
Breast, w/o skin, ground	4 oz.	34	0	1
Dark meat, w/o skin, roasted	4 oz.	32	0	8
Premium sliced deli breast	3 oz.	20	0	1
Turkey roll, light meat	2 slices	10	0	1
Veal				
Loin, w/o skin, roasted	4 oz.	29	0	8
Sirloin, w/o skin, roasted	4 oz.	30	0	7
Shoulder, w/o skin, roasted	4 oz.	29	0	7

Carbohydrate Sources

Glycemic Rating: L = low, M = medium, M/H = medium/high, H = high, VH = very high

FOOD	SERVING SIZE	GLYCEMIC RATING	PROTEIN GRAMS	CARB. GRAMS	FAT GRAMS
Fruits					
Apple	1 medium	M	0	21	0
Applesauce (unsweetened)	1/2 cup	M	0	14	0
Apricots, fresh	3 fruits	M/H	1	12	0
Apricots, water packed	1/2 cup	M/H	1	8	0
Avocado, raw	1/4	L	1	3	8
Banana	1 each	H	1	26	1
Blackberries, raw	1/2 cup	L	1	9	0
Blueberries, raw	1/2 cup	L	1	10	0
Cantaloupe	1/2 melon	L	2	22	1
Cherries	1/2 cup	L	1	12	1
Cranberry sauce	1/4 cup	H	0	27	0
Dates	2 dates	H	0	12	0
Figs, raw	1 medium	H	0	10	0
Fruit cocktail, water packed	1/2 cup	M	0	11	0
Grapefruit	1/2 fruit	L	1	10	0
Grapes	10 fruits	M	0	5	0
Guava, cubed	1/2 cup	M	1	14	1
Honeydew melon	1/10 melon	L	1	12	0
Kiwi fruit	1 medium	L	1	11	0
Mango, cubed	1/2 cup	M/H	1	14	0
Nectarine	1 fruit	M	1	16	0
Lemon or Lime juice	1 Tbsp.	M	0	1	0
Orange	1 fruit	M	1	16	0
Papaya, cubed	1/2 cup	H	0	11	0
Peach, fresh, 2 1/2"	1 fruit	L	0	10	0
Peaches, canned/water	1/2 cup	L	0	8	0
Pear, fresh, 2 1/2"	1 fruit	L	0	25	0
Pears, canned/water	1/2 cup	L	0	10	0
Pineapple, fresh	1 cup	L	1	20	0
Plum, raw, 2 1/8"	1 fruit	L	0	9	0
Prunes, dried	2 fruits	M	0	11	0
Raisins	1/4 cup	H	1	33	0
Raspberries, raw	1/2 cup	L	0	7	0
Strawberries	1 cup	L	1	11	0
Tangerine	1 fruit	M	0	9	0
Watermelon, cubed	1 cup	M	1	12	0
Vegetables					
Alfalfa sprouts	1 cup	L	1	1	0
Artichoke, cooked	1 medium	L	4	14	0
Asparagus	1 cup	L	7	8	0
Bamboo shoots	1/2 cup	L	2	4	0
Bean sprouts	1/2 cup	L	4	7	0
Beets, canned	1/2 cup	M	1	6	0
Bok choy	1/2 cup	L	0	1	0
Broccoli	1 cup	L	6	12	1
Butternut squash	1/2 cup	M	1	11	0
Brussels sprouts	1 cup	L	6	20	1
Cabbage, shredded	1 cup	L	3	12	0

FOOD	SERVING SIZE	GLYCEMIC RATING	PROTEIN GRAMS	CARB. GRAMS	FAT GRAMS
Vegetables, continued					
Carrots, cooked	1 cup	H	2	23	0
Cauliflower	1 cup	L	4	11	0
Chili pepper, raw	1/4 cup	L	0	2	0
Celery, raw	1 stalk	L	0	2	0
Cucumber, sliced	1/2 cup	L	0	2	0
Collards, boiled	1/2 cup	L	1	4	0
Corn	1/2 cup	H	3	21	1
Corn on the cob	1/2 ear	H	2	14	0
Eggplant, cubed	1 cup	L	1	7	0
Endive, raw	1/2 cup	L	0	1	0
Green beans (snap)	1 cup	L	2	8	0
Green pepper	1/2 cup	L	0	3	0
Hummus	1/4 cup	L	3	13	6
Kale, boiled	1/2 cup	L	1	4	0
Leeks, raw	1/4 cup	L	1	4	0
Lentils, boiled	1/2 cup	M	9	20	0
Lettuce, Iceberg	1 cup	L	2	5	0
Butterhead	5 leaves	L	0	1	0
Romaine	1 cup	L	3	5	0
Mushrooms, raw	1/2 cup	L	1	2	0
Mustard greens, raw	1/2 cup	L	1	1	0
Onion, raw	1/2 cup	L	1	7	0
Okra, boiled	1/2 cup	L	1	6	0
Parsnips, boiled	1/2 cup	H	1	15	0
Parsley, chopped	1 Tbsp.	L	0	1	0
Peas, green	1/2 cup	M	4	11	0
Pickles, cucumber dill	1 each	L	0	3	0
Pickles, sweet	1 each	H	0	11	0
Poi	1/2 cup	H	1	33	0
Red radish, raw	4 each	L	0	1	0
Salsa	1 oz.	L	0	2	0
Sauerkraut	1/2 cup	L	0	4	0
Snow peas, raw	1/2 cup	L	2	6	0
Spinach, raw	1/2 cup	L	1	1	0
Summer squash, boiled	1/2 cup	M	1	4	0
Swiss chard, raw	1/2 cup	L	0	1	0
Tempeh	1/2 cup	L	16	14	6
Tofu, extra-firm	4 oz.	L	12	1	6
Tofu, soft	4 oz.	L	8	2	5
Tomato	1 medium	L	1	6	0
Tomato sauce (no sugar)	1/2 cup	L	2	9	0
Turnip, boiled	1/2 cup	L	1	6	0
Turnip greens, boiled	1/2 cup	L	1	3	0
Zucchini, raw	1/2 cup	L	1	2	0
Breads/Starches					
Bagel, plain	1 each	H	8	38	1
Bagel, raisin/cinn.	1 each	H	7	40	1
Biscuit, buttermilk	1 each	H	2	17	6
Bread crumbs	1/2 cup	H	7	39	3
Bread sticks 7 5/8"	1 stick	H	1	7	1
Bread, white	1 slice	H	2	12	1
Bread, wheat	1 slice	H	3	12	1
Bread, reduced calorie	1 slice	H	2	10	1
Bread, rye (pumpernickel)	1 slice	H	3	15	1

FOOD	SERVING SIZE	GLYCEMIC RATING	PROTEIN GRAMS	CARB. GRAMS	FAT GRAMS
Bread/Starches, continued					
Bread, French, 4.75 x 4"	1 slice	H	4	26	2
Buns, hamburger/hot dog	1 each	H	4	22	2
Buns, reduced calorie	1 each	H	4	18	1
Cornbread	1 slice	H	4	29	6
Croissant	1 medium	H	4	19	19
Croutons, plain	1 oz.	H	1	3	0
Croutons, seasoned	1 oz.	H	1	3	1
Dinner roll	1 each	H	3	15	1
English muffin	1 each	H	5	25	1
Pita pocket 6.5 dia.	1 each	H	6	35	2
Buckwheat, dried	2 oz.	M	7	41	1
Bulgur wheat, cooked	1/2 cup	M	10	58	1
Grits, cooked	1/2 cup	H	2	16	0
Cornmeal, dry	1/4 cup	H	2	23	1
Couscous, cooked	1/2 cup	H	3	21	0
Egg noodles, cooked	1 cup	H	8	40	3
Flour, wheat, all purpose	1 cup	H	16	87	2
Flour, rye flour	1 cup	H	9	82	1
Hominy, canned	1/2 cup	M	1	12	1
Kashi, cooked	1/2 cup	M	6	30	3
Macaroni, cooked	1 cup	M	6	40	1
Millet, cooked	1/2 cup	H	4	28	
Muffins, bran	1 medium	H	3	23	5
Muffins, blueberry	1 medium	H	3	27	4
Noodles, cooked	1 cup	M	8	40	2
Oat bran, cooked	1/2 cup	H	3	12	1
Oatmeal, cooked	1 cup	M	6	25	2
Pancakes 4" each	1 each	H	2	13	3
Pasta, cooked	1 cup	M	12	56	2
Popcorn, air popped	3 cup	VH	2	15	0
Potato, baked	1 large	VH	5	49	0
Potato, mashed	1/2 cup	VH	2	19	1
Potato, red, new	3 small	M	2	14	0
Rice cakes, plain	1 each	VH	1	7	0
Rice, brown, cooked	1 cup	M/H	4	46	2
Rice, white, cooked	1 cup	M/H	5	57	0
Spaghetti, wheat	1 cup	M/H	7	38	1
Sweet potato	1/2 each	M/H	1	14	0
Stuffing, prepared	1/2 cup	H	3	22	9
Taco shell	1 medium	M	1	8	3
Tortilla, corn 7" dia.	1 item	M	1	12	1
Tortilla, flour 7" dia.	1 item	H	3	20	2
Waffles, 4" square	1 item	H	2	14	3
Yam, cooked	1/2 cup	M/H	1	19	0
Beans					
Baked beans	1/2 cup	M/H	6	26	1
Black beans, boiled	1/2 cup	M	8	20	1
Kidney beans, boiled	1/2 cup	M	8	20	1
Lima beans	1/2 cup	M	7	20	0
Navy beans, boiled	1/2 cup	M	8	24	1
Pinto beans, boiled	1/2 cup	M	8	24	1
Refried beans	1/2 cup	M	8	24	1
White beans, boiled	1/2 cup	M	9	23	0

FOOD	SERVING SIZE	PROTEIN GRAMS	CARB. GRAMS	FAT GRAMS
Nuts and Seeds				
Almonds, raw	1 Tbsp.	3	3	8
Almond butter	1 Tbsp.	4	4	9
Cashews, raw	1 Tbsp.	3	5	7
Peanuts, raw	1 Tbsp.	4	3	7
Peanut butter	1 Tbsp.	4	3	7
Pecans, raw	1 Tbsp.	1	3	10
Pine nuts, raw	1 Tbsp.	4	2	8
Pistachios, raw	1 Tbsp.	3	4	7
Pumpkin seeds, raw	1 Tbsp.	4	3	7
Sesame seeds, raw	1 Tbsp.	3	3	8
Sunflower seeds, raw	1 Tbsp.	3	3	8
Walnuts, raw	1 Tbsp.	2	3	9
Fats and Oils				
Butter,	1 Tbsp.	0	0	11
Butter, whipped	1 Tbsp.	0	0	8
Canola oil	1 Tbsp.	0	0	14
Cream cheese, Philly light	2 Tbsp.	3	2	5
Mayonnaise, full-fat	1 Tbsp.	0	0	11
Mayonnaise, low-fat	1 Tbsp.	0	1	5
Flax seed oil	1 Tbsp.	0	0	14
Olive oil	1 Tbsp.	0	0	14
Olives, green, pitted	5 medium	0	0	3
Olives, Greek style	5 medium	0	0	3
Peanut oil	1 Tbsp.	0	0	14
Safflower oil	1 Tbsp.	0	0	14
Sour cream, lite	2 Tbsp.	2	2	2
Wheat germ oil	1 Tbsp.	0	0	14

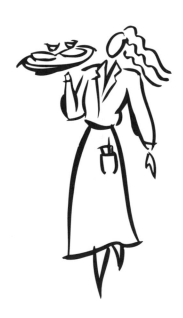

Restaurants, Prepared Foods, and Fast Food Guide

Chapter 12

EAT OUT, BUT EAT SMART

Once reserved for special occasions, restaurant eating has now become an everyday event for many Americans. More and more restaurants are attempting to offer healthy alternatives for their customers. However, they still bombard us with meals high in carbohydrate, fat, cholesterol, and salt. The trick to balancing a dining experience is remembering to apply the *40-30-30 Fat-Burning Nutrition* principles—wherever you are.

If you tend to overeat in restaurants, avoid complete dinners with several courses and the all-you-can-eat buffets and smorgasbords. Instead, order a la carte. This gives you more control over portions. When baskets of chips or bread and butter on the table are too much of a temptation, simply ask that they be removed.

Order appetizers that are high in protein such as shrimp or crab cocktail, smoked salmon, oysters, or chicken skewers. Begin your meal with a broth-based soup or a green salad, both of which are very low in carbohydrate. Remember, you have the right to request your meal be prepared to suit your taste and needs. Most restaurants will be happy to make adjustments to ensure a satisfied customer.

Here are a few basic guidelines to remember when you eat out:

- Many restaurant meals contain large portions of carbohydrate and small portions of protein. Carbohydrate is relatively inexpensive–especially the starchy carbohydrates like pasta, potatoes, rice, and bread–while protein is relatively expensive. Always ask what comes with your meal so you are aware of what you will be eating. Order extra vegetables and include a green salad.

- If you will be having an alcoholic beverage with dinner, either have it served <u>with</u> your meal, or drink it before dinner with a protein appetizer.

- If you are planning to have dessert, limit or eliminate the starches (potato, rice, pasta, and bread) in your meal and increase the vegetables and salad. Eat only half of the dessert or share it with a friend.

- If you have a meal or special occasion where you eat too much or the wrong ratio, don't become completely discouraged. *40-30-30 Fat-Burning Nutrition* works because you can maximize your body's ability to burn stored body fat for energy, every time you eat. If you get off track, simply get back on track at your next meal.

With a few adjustments, you can eat out almost anywhere and follow the *40-30-30 Fat-Burning Nutrition* principles to maximize fat burning. Listed are examples from different types of restaurants.

CONTINENTAL (EUROPEAN CUISINE)

Most continental cuisine can be very balanced. Limit or avoid bread. Choose a grilled piece of protein with vegetables, a small serving of starchy carbohydrate, and a green salad.

CONTINENTAL MEAL EXAMPLES:

Grilled Fish or Chicken with a Small Caesar Salad

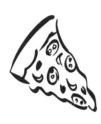

- Grilled chicken breast or fish
- Vegetables, steamed
- Choose only one starch with your meal. If you are having bread pass on the potatoes, rice, or pasta and ask for extra vegetables.
- Caesar salad
- Mineral water with lemon

Gourmet Pizza

- Have a small, thin-crust gourmet pizza with grilled chicken and vegetables plus a large dinner salad. The pizza crust contains sufficient carbohydrates, so avoid any additional bread or dessert.

MEXICAN

Mexican food is typically very high in fat: cheese, avocados, refried beans, and sour cream. It also contains the worst kind of carbohydrate: starchy and fried. But, with the right choices, Mexican food can be very balanced. Choose sizzling fajitas and have only one of the starches: tortilla, rice, beans, or chips. If choosing chips, have them with your meal. Use only small servings of added fat and top with generous portions of tomatoes, salsa, and lettuce.

MEXICAN MEAL EXAMPLE:

Sizzling Fajitas (chicken, fish, beef, or pork)

- Chicken fajitas
- Two flour tortillas
- Ask for extra vegetables and no rice or beans.
- 1-2 T. guacamole or sour cream
- Salsa, tomatoes, and lettuce
- Iced tea

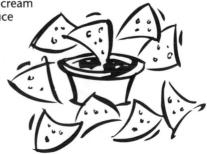

ITALIAN

Italian cuisine can be very high in starchy carbohydrate (pasta and bread), high in fat (olive oil and cheese), and low in protein. It is one of our favorites and can be yours too with a few adjustments. Choose a lean protein entree with vegetables and a salad. Include a small side order of pasta served with a tomato-based sauce and skip the bread. If drinking wine, cut back on the pasta.

ITALIAN MEAL EXAMPLE:

Lemon Chicken with Tomato Fettuccine
- Lemon chicken
- Fettuccine with red sauce
- Vegetables
- Dinner salad with olive oil and vinegar dressing
- Mineral water (S. Pellagrino)
- 1 glass red wine

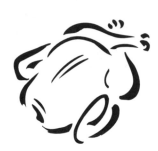

JAPANESE

Japanese cuisine is one of the most balanced, but watch out for eating too much rice and not getting enough protein. Avoid batter-fried tempura and choose grilled fish or chicken with vegetables and a small amount of steamed rice.

JAPANESE MEAL EXAMPLE:

Grilled Teriyaki Chicken with Steamed Vegetables
- Teriyaki chicken
- Steamed vegetables
- Rice (1/2 to 1 cup)
- Small salad
- Hot tea

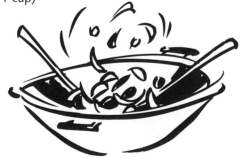

CHINESE

Chinese cuisine can be very high in fat, sodium, and carbohydrate. The best choices are grilled or stir-fried chicken or fish with steamed vegetables and limited quantities of rice.

CHINESE MEAL EXAMPLE:

Stir-Fried Chicken and Broccoli

- Chicken
- Rice (1/2 to 1 cup)
- Hot tea
- 1 fortune cookie
- Broccoli
- Sweet and sour soup
- Water

AMERICAN DINERS AND COFFEE SHOPS

Basic American cuisine can be very high in fat and starchy carbohydrate (usually lots of bread, cheese, fatty sauces, and gravies). Our recommendation for lunch or dinner would be the same as for Continental. Breakfast can be especially difficult, but with a little effort, it can be done. Choose lean protein, only one starchy carbohydrate, and fruit.

AMERICAN DINERS AND COFFEE SHOPS MEAL EXAMPLE:

Poached Eggs with Toast and Grapefruit

- 3 poached eggs (discard 2 yolks)
- 1 slice toast with jam
- 1/2 grapefruit
- Coffee or tea, decaffeinated
- Water

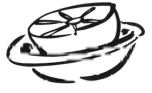

DELI

Delis generally provide quality protein but can be too high in fat. Choose a lean protein sandwich without cheese and use mayonnaise sparingly. Skip the potato and pasta salads that are loaded with fat and carbohydrate, and have a small piece of fruit or a side salad or cole slaw.

DELI MEAL EXAMPLE:

Turkey on Rye

- Sliced turkey breast, (3-4 ozs.)
- Two slices of rye or sourdough bread
- Lettuce and tomato
- Mayonnaise (use sparingly) and/or mustard
- 1 dill pickle
- 1 small piece of fruit or slaw
- Mineral water, iced tea, or diet soda

PREPARED FOODS

There are many low-fat prepared, canned, and frozen foods. Most of them are high in carbohydrate and low in protein. Just like in the restaurants, the prepackaged food manufacturers load up on the less expensive carbohydrate and cut back on the more expensive protein. Prepared foods can also be very high in sodium, so read the labels carefully. Avoid high-sodium meals if you are on a low-sodium diet.

Below are some examples of prepared foods that can be used with *40-30-30 Fat-Burning Nutrition*. Each meal should contain approximately 40 percent of the total calories coming from carbohydrate, 30 percent from protein, and 30 percent from fat. If a meal is too low in fat, add a side salad with a quality salad dressing.

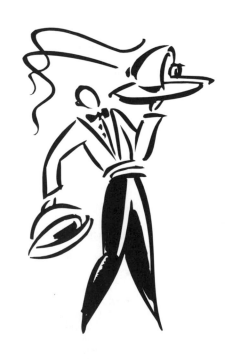

Prepared Food Guide

FROZEN FOODS

FOOD	CALORIES	CARB. GRAMS	PROTEIN GRAMS	FAT GRAMS
Armour Classics				
• Mesquite Chicken and Noodles	230	23	19	7
• Oriental Chicken	180	24	18	1
Healthy Choice				
• Chicken and Pasta Divan	300	41	25	4
• Glazed Chicken	220	27	21	3
• Honey Mustard Chicken	250	37	24	3
• Mandarin Chicken	240	35	21	2
• Chicken Fettuccine	240	29	22	4
• Chicken with Peanut Sauce	280	31	29	5
• Turkey Dinner	270	30	27	4
• Chicken Fajitas	200	24	17	5
Lean Cuisine				
• Chicken Cacciatore w/Vermicelli	280	31	22	7
• Chicken Italian w/Fettuccine	270	33	22	6
• Chicken Marsala w/Vegetables	180	13	22	4
• Glazed Chicken w/Vegetable Rice	250	42	21	7
• Turkey with Stuffing	270	27	19	9
• Turkey with Rice Pilaf	230	24	17	6
• Turkey Dijon	210	20	20	6
The Budget Gourmet				
• Beef Stroganoff	260	27	19	10
• Herb Chicken with Fettuccine	240	30	21	6
• Mesquite Chicken	250	33	23	6
• Pot Roast	230	25	19	7
• Turkey Dinner	250	31	21	6
Tyson Healthy Portion				
• Chicken Marinara, Healthy Portion	340	37	31	7
• Glazed Chicken	240	29	22	4
• Grilled Chicken	220	22	26	3
• Herb Chicken, Healthy Portion	340	43	32	4
• Italian Dinner, Healthy Portion	310	38	30	4
• Mesquite Chicken, Healthy Portion	330	38	34	5
Weight Watchers				
• Chicken Fettuccine	280	25	22	9
• Chicken and Noodles	240	25	19	7
• Lasagna	270	29	24	6
• Imperial Chicken	200	25	18	3
• Italian Lasagna	290	29	28	7
• Cordon Bleu	170	19	15	5
• Chicken Fajitas	210	24	17	5

SOUPS

FOOD	CALORIES	CARB. GRAMS	PROTEIN GRAMS	FAT GRAMS
Campbell's				
• Chunky Beef	160	15	13	5
• Chunky Chicken Noodle	170	16	12	6
• Home Cooking Chicken Noodle	110	10	11	3
• Home Cooking Vegetable Beef	120	15	12	5
Healthy Choice				
• Beef and Potato	120	16	11	1
• Chunky Beef Vegetable	110	14	10	1
Progresso				
• Beef Barley	130	15	12	4
• Beef Noodle	160	17	15	4
• Beef Minestrone	160	16	13	5
• Beef Vegetable	140	14	14	3
• Chicken Barley	130	11	12	3
• Chicken Noodle Soup	80	10	7	2
• Hearty Chicken	130	11	12	4
• Home Style Chicken	110	11	10	3
• Manhattan Clam Chowder	120	13	13	2
• Tomato, Beef with Rotini	160	17	12	5

CHILIS

FOOD	CALORIES	CARB. GRAMS	PROTEIN GRAMS	FAT GRAMS
Hain				
• Spicy with Chicken	130	19	11	2
Healthy Choice				
• Spicy Turkey	210	26	17	5
• Turkey with Beans	200	20	18	5

Prepared Food Tips:

1. If a commercially prepared meal is too high in carbohydrate and too low in protein, add a quality, low-fat protein like cottage cheese or sliced chicken or turkey.

2. If a meal is too low in fat, have a small salad with 1-2 T. of salad dressing.

3. If a meal is too low in carbohydrate, add some fresh fruit or vegetables.

4. Canned and prepared foods can contain high amounts of sodium. Always read the labels to be aware of sodium content if you are on a low-sodium diet.

LIGHT, SANDWICHES

FOOD	CALORIES	CARB. GRAMS	PROTEIN GRAMS	FAT GRAMS
Arby's				
• Roast Beef Deluxe	294	33	18	10
• Roast Chicken Deluxe	276	33	24	7
• Roast Turkey Deluxe	260	33	20	6
Burger King				
• BK Broiler Chicken Sandwich	280	29	20	10
Carl's Jr.				
• Charbroiled Chicken Sandwich	310	34	25	6
Dairy Queen				
• Grilled Chicken Sandwich	300	33	25	8
Hardee's				
• Grilled Chicken Sandwich	310	34	24	9
Jack In The Box				
• Chicken Fajita Pita	292	29	24	8
McDonalds				
• McGrilled Chicken Sandwich	250	33	24	3
Taco Bell				
• Light Taco	140	13	11	5
• Light Taco Supreme	160	14	13	5
• Light Soft Taco	180	19	13	5
• Light Soft Taco Supreme	200	23	14	5
• Light Taco Salad w/o chips	330	35	30	9
Wendy's				
• Grilled Chicken Sandwich	290	35	24	7
• Chili (small)	190	21	19	6
• Chili (large)	290	31	28	9

Special Fast Food Tips:

1. Avoid all fried foods.
2. Avoid sugar-containing beverages. Have water, iced tea, or diet soda.
3. You can always include a small green salad and use low-fat salad dressing or small amounts of full-fat salad dressing.
4. Plain soft chicken tacos or grilled fish tacos and burritos without rice or beans are excellent choices at most Mexican fast food restaurants.
5. Most grilled or roasted chicken sandwiches without cheese will be balanced.
6. Remember, try not to make eating in fast-food restaurants a daily habit. Take the time to prepare more nutritious meals.

Are There Fat-Burning Supplements?

Chapter 13

There are literally thousands of pills, powders, herbal products, stimulants, and many other supplements that claim to be fat burners, but *nothing* is as powerful in burning fat as is minimizing insulin and elevating glucagon. The most powerful tool for burning fat is the food you eat or, more specifically, the *ratio* of the carbohydrate, protein, and fat in your meals.

> **Caution**: Stimulant supplements can actually elevate insulin and prevent you from maximizing fat burning. In general, we recommend you avoid all stimulant-based supplements.

Food is the body's most powerful fat burner. However, we have found a few products that can be very useful to you as food supplements. Listed below are products you can use with *40-30-30 Fat-Burning Nutrition*.

Protein Powders. It's easy to eat too many carbohydrates and sometimes hard to eat adequate amounts of protein. Protein powders can be a simple, economical, convenient, and tasty way to add quality protein to your diet.

When shopping for a protein powder, make sure it contains predominately protein with very little carbohydrate or fat. Add your own carbohydrate and fat, such as fruit and nuts, to make a balanced shake.

Use a 40-30-30 protein shake when you don't have time to make a meal. Protein powders can also be added to many high-carbohydrate foods to make them more balanced.

You will find many different varieties of protein powders such as egg white, egg and milk combination, soy, and whey. Whey protein is the new generation of protein powders and has many advantages over other protein powders. It is very high in protein, contains very little fat or carbohydrate, has little or no taste, mixes instantly, and can be used in cooking or baking. It also has a very good amino acid profile.

Multi Vitamin and Mineral. We recommend using a highly absorbable multiple vitamin and mineral complex as a form of nutritional insurance to add to your well-balanced meals.

Chromium. Chromium is a trace mineral that is a co-factor to insulin and is needed for insulin metabolism. Without chromium, your body needs more insulin to function properly. With normal levels of chromium, you need less insulin. However, chromium will not work, no matter how much you take, unless you first control the ratio of the foods you eat which ultimately controls the release of insulin.

Nutrition Bars. Nutrition bars can be one of the best or worst food supplements for burning fat, depending on the ratio of the carbohydrate, protein, and fat they contain. Most nutrition bars are extremely high in carbohydrates, increase blood sugar, and elevate insulin levels minimizing your ability to burn fat.

At the BioSyn Human Performance Center, we used *40-30-30 Fat-Burning Nutrition* along with a nutrition bar that had an exact 40-30-30 ratio of carbohydrate, protein and fat. It was used to substitute a meal or snack when it was difficult to make a balanced meal. Half a bar was also used 30 minutes before exercising and half after.

We recommend using a 40-30-30 nutrition bar that contains a blend of high quality protein sources to ensure a sufficient ratio of the essential amino acids. It should also contain a blend of low, medium, and high glycemic carbohydrate sources and contain "good" fat sources. We also recommend the bar contains vitamins and minerals including antioxidants and chromium.

Remember, the most powerful tool for burning fat is the food you eat, or more specifically the *ratio* of the food you eat! Food supplements can be useful in helping you burn stored body fat for energy, but not nearly as powerful as *40-30-30 Fat-Burning Nutrition.* Supplement your diet with quality vitamins and minerals and use a 40-30-30 meal replacement bar when you don't have time to make a balanced meal, as a healthy fat-burning snack, or before you exercise.

Note: Always consult with your doctor first before starting any supplement, weight-loss, or fitness program.

Appendix

Studies show that subjects on a weekly diet program lost 50 percent more weight, snacked less, and bought more fruits and vegetables when given a detailed meal planner and grocery list to follow. By reviewing the Sample Starter Meal Planners provided in Chapter 8, *"Putting It All Together,"* you can determine the foods you will need to have on hand. Make copies of the grocery list and use it to plan your weekly meals. You may want to use the Food Value Guide in Chapter 11 and Prepared Foods from Chapter 12 for additional food choices. Plan one week at a time.

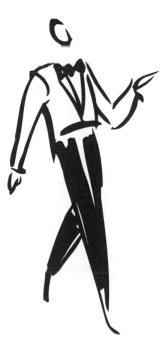

FBN 40-30-30 QUICK-START SHOPPING LIST

Review the meals in this book and choose your favorites to prepare your shopping list.

Nutritional Supplement Products
- ☐ 40-30-30 Nutrition Bar
- ☐ Whey Protein Powder

Carbohydrate 40%

FRUITS
- ☐ apples
- ☐ bananas
- ☐ grapes
- ☐ oranges
- ☐ peaches, fresh or frozen
- ☐ pears
- ☐ pineapple, fresh or canned
- ☐ orange juice
- ☐ strawberries, fresh or frozen
- ☐ mixed berries, frozen
- ☐ plum
- ☐ kiwi
- _____
- _____
- _____
- _____

VEGETABLES
- ☐ asparagus
- ☐ broccoli
- ☐ red bell pepper
- ☐ celery
- ☐ green beans
- ☐ green bell pepper
- ☐ lettuce
- ☐ onion, sweet
- ☐ spinach
- ☐ tomatoes
- ☐ cabbage
- ☐ cucumber
- ☐ lettuce, romaine
- ☐ snow peas
- ☐ mushrooms
- _____
- _____

STARCHES*
- ☐ bagel
- ☐ brown rice
- ☐ bread**
- ☐ bran muffin
- ☐ pasta
- ☐ pita bread
- ☐ oatmeal
- ☐ red "new" potatoes
- ☐ taco shells
- ☐ tortilla, flour
- ☐ granola, small amount
- ☐ All Bran cereal
- ☐ English muffins
- ☐ pinto beans
- ☐ corn on the cob
- _____
- _____

Protein (low-fat) 30%

- ☐ 2% cottage cheese
- ☐ milk, non fat
- ☐ eggs
- ☐ cheddar cheese, low-fat
- ☐ Swiss cheese, low-fat
- ☐ ground sirloin, x-lean
- _____
- _____

- ☐ deli turkey, sliced
- ☐ yogurt
- ☐ salmon steak
- ☐ Albacore tuna (in water)
- ☐ red snapper
- _____
- _____

- ☐ Canadian bacon
- ☐ chicken breast
- ☐ tempeh
- ☐ tofu
- ☐ Boca burgers
- _____
- _____

Fat 30%

- ☐ almonds, raw
- ☐ mayonnaise
- ☐ salad dressing, low-fat
- ☐ salad dressing, full-fat
- _____

- ☐ avocado
- ☐ olive oil
- ☐ sour cream
- ☐ coleslaw dressing
- _____

- ☐ macadamia nuts, raw
- ☐ vegetable oil
- ☐ cream cheese, low-fat, whipped
- _____

Miscellaneous

- ☐ honey
- ☐ crystalline fructose
- ☐ pickle relish, sweet
- _____
- _____

- ☐ soy sauce
- ☐ salsa, mild to hot
- ☐ pizza sauce
- _____
- _____

- ☐ pasta sauce***
- ☐ barbecue sauce
- ☐ meat marinade
- _____
- _____

*Avoid if following the Fat-Flush meals.   **Reduced-calorie if using "A"   ***Sugar- and fat-free

Tracking Your Results

This book belongs to:

NAME: _____

ADDRESS: _____

CITY, STATE, ZIP: _____

PHONE: _____

DATE STARTED: _____ / _____ / _____

Track results by recording your weight, body fat percentage (if known), and your waist measurement.

Check Meal Planner Used	A ☐	B ☐	C ☐	D ☐

WEEK 1: DATE _____ WEIGHT _____ % BODY FAT _____ WAIST _____

WEEK 2: DATE _____ WEIGHT _____ % BODY FAT _____ WAIST _____

WEEK 3: DATE _____ WEIGHT _____ % BODY FAT _____ WAIST _____

WEEK 4: DATE _____ WEIGHT _____ % BODY FAT _____ WAIST _____

WEEK 5: DATE _____ WEIGHT _____ % BODY FAT _____ WAIST _____

WEEK 6: DATE _____ WEIGHT _____ % BODY FAT _____ WAIST _____

Check Meal Planner Used	A ☐	B ☐	C ☐	D ☐

WEEK 7: DATE _____ WEIGHT _____ % BODY FAT _____ WAIST _____

WEEK 8: DATE _____ WEIGHT _____ % BODY FAT _____ WAIST _____

WEEK 9: DATE _____ WEIGHT _____ % BODY FAT _____ WAIST _____

WEEK 10: DATE _____ WEIGHT _____ % BODY FAT _____ WAIST _____

WEEK 11: DATE _____ WEIGHT _____ % BODY FAT _____ WAIST _____

WEEK 12: DATE _____ WEIGHT _____ % BODY FAT _____ WAIST _____

Check Meal Planner Used	A ☐	B ☐	C ☐	D ☐

WEEK 13: DATE _____ WEIGHT _____ % BODY FAT _____ WAIST _____

WEEK 14: DATE _____ WEIGHT _____ % BODY FAT _____ WAIST _____

WEEK 15: DATE _____ WEIGHT _____ % BODY FAT _____ WAIST _____

WEEK 16: DATE _____ WEIGHT _____ % BODY FAT _____ WAIST _____

WEEK 17: DATE _____ WEIGHT _____ % BODY FAT _____ WAIST _____

40-30-30 FBN PROPORTION CHART

40-30-30 Fat-Burning Nutrition is simply a more balanced approach to nutrition. Listed is a 40-30-30 Proportion Chart. You can use this chart as a guide to help you determine what the 40-30-30 ratios should be when using grams and/or calories.

Gram Proportions

40% Carb. (In Grams)	30% Protein (In Grams)	30% Fat (In Grams)
7	5	2.2
13	10	4.4
20	15	6.6
27	20	8.8
33	25	11.1
40	30	13.3
47	35	15.6
53	40	17.8

Calorie Proportions

Calories	40% Carb. Cal. - Grams	30% Protein Cal. - Grams	30% Fat Cal. - Grams
50	20 - 5	15 - 3.6	15 - 1.7
100	40 - 10	30 - 7.5	30 - 3.3
150	60 - 15	45 - 11.3	45 - 5
200	80 - 20	60 - 15	60 - 6.7
250	100 - 25	75 - 18.8	75 - 8.3
300	120 - 30	90 - 22.5	90 - 10
350	140 - 35	105 - 26.3	105 - 11.7
400	160 - 40	120 - 30	120 - 13.3
450	180 - 45	135 - 33.8	135 - 15
500	200 - 50	150 - 37.5	150 - 16.7

Total Daily Calorie Proportions

Calories	40% Carb. Cal. - Grams	30% Protein Cal. - Grams	30% Fat Cal. - Grams
1000	400 - 100	300 - 75	300 - 33.3
1250	500 - 125	375 - 93.8	375 - 41.7
1500	600 - 150	450 - 112.5	450 - 50
1750	700 - 175	525 - 131.3	525 - 58.3
2000	800 - 200	600 - 150	600 - 66.7
2500	1000 - 250	750 - 187.5	750 - 83.3

■ Carbohydrate should be 1/3 more than protein, or protein x 1.33 = carbohydrate. Each 1 gram of carbohydrate and protein contains 4 calories. To calculate carbohydrate and protein calories, multiply grams by 4.

■ Fat calories and protein calories are the same (30%). Because fat has 9 calories per gram, the fat grams will be less than half of the protein grams. To calculate fat calories multiply grams by 9.

RECOMMENDED READING LIST

1. Anderson, L., et al. *Nutrition in Health and Disease*. Philadelphia, PA: J. B. Lippincott, 1982

2. Ensminger, A., et al. *Foods and Nutrition Encyclopedia*. 2nd ed. Boca Raton, FL: CRC Press, 1994

3. Latifi, R., *Amino Acids in Critical Care and Cancer*. George Town, TX: R. G. Landes, 1994

4. Mills, M., et al. *David and Passmore Human Nutrition and Dietetics*. 8th ed. New York, NY: Churchchill Livingstone, 1986

5. *Modern Nutrition in Health and Disease*. 8th ed. Shils, M et al., ed. Malvern, PA: Lea & Febiger, 1994

6. Netzer, C., *The Complete Book of Food Counts*. New York, NY: Bantam Doubleday Dell, 1994

7. *Nutritional Biochemistry and Metabolism with Clinical Applications*. Linder, M.ed. New York, NY: Elsevier, 1985

8. Paige, D., *Clinical Nutrition*. 2nd ed. St. Louis, MO: C.V. Mosby, 1988

9. Pemberton, C., et al. *Mayo Clinic Diet Manual*. 6th ed. Saint Louis, MO: C.V. Mosby, 1988

10. *Recommended Dietary Allowances*. Washington, DC: National Academy Press, 1989

11. Robinson, C., et al. *Basic Nutrition and Diet Therapy*. 7th ed. New York, NY: Macmillian, 1993

12. Snetselaar, L., *Nutrition Counseling Skills*. 2nd ed. Rockville, NY: Aspen, 1989

13. *The Surgeon General's Report on Nutrition and Health*. U.S. Department of Health and Human Services.

14. Werbach, M., *Nutritional Influences on Illness*. New Canaan, CT: Keats, 1988

15. Whitney, E., et al. *Understanding Nutrition*. 5th ed. St. Paul, MN: West, 1990

16. Williams, M., *Nutritional Aspects of Human Physical and Athletic Performance*. 2nd ed. Springfield, IL: Charles C.Thomas, 1985

17. Williams, S., et al. *Nutrition and Diet Therapy*. 7th ed. St. Louis, MO: Mosby, 1993

RECOMMENDED READING LIST, CONTINUED

Journals

18. *The American Journal Of Clinical Nutrition.*

19. *Diabetes.* A Journal of The American Diabetes Association.

20. *Hormone Research.*

21. *JAMA.* The Journal of the American Medical Association.

22. *The Journal of Clinical Endocrinology and Metabolism.*

23. *European Journal of Clinical Nutrition.*

24. *International Journal for Vitamin and Nutrition Research.*

25. *The Journal of Lipid Research.*

26. *International Journal of Obesity.*

27. *International Journal of Peptide and Protein Research.*

28. *Journal of the American College of Nutrition.*

29. *Journal of the American Dietetic Association.*

30. *The Journal of Nutrition.*

31. *The Lancet.*

32. *The New England Journal of Medicine.*

33. *Nutrition and Cancer.*

34. *Nutrition Research.*

35. *Nutrition Today.*

36. *Progress in Cardiovascular Disease.*

37. *Prostaglandins.*

38. *Prostaglandins, Leukotrienes and Essential Fatty Acids.*